Atkins Diet Book 2023 - 2024

Rapid Weight Loss, Burn Fat, and the Simpler, Faster Path to a Low-Carb Lifestyle – Achieve Weight Loss Without Sacrifice

By
Helen Munoz

Atkins diet book

Copyright

Disclaimer:

The information provided in this book is for educational and informational purposes only. It is not intended to be a substitute for professional medical advice, diagnosis, or treatment. Always seek the advice of your physician or other qualified health provider with any questions you may have regarding a medical condition. The author and publisher of this book are not responsible for any specific health or allergy needs that may require medical supervision and are not liable for any damages or negative consequences arising from the use of the information contained herein. The reader assumes full responsibility for consulting a qualified health professional regarding health conditions and before starting a new diet or health program.

About the author

Helen Munoz, the insightful mind behind the Atkins Diet Book 2023-2024, is a dedicated advocate for holistic health and wellness. With a passion for empowering individuals on their journey to a healthier lifestyle, Helen brings a unique blend of experience and expertise to the world of dieting.

Helen's educational background includes a degree in Nutrition Science, providing her with a solid foundation in understanding the intricate relationship between food, metabolism, and overall well-being. Her commitment to ongoing learning ensures that her insights are rooted in the latest advancements in the field.

Having navigated her personal wellness journey, Helen understands the challenges that individuals face in achieving sustainable weight loss. Her approach emphasizes a low-carb lifestyle, incorporating the principles of the Atkins diet for effective and enjoyable weight management.

Beyond her academic pursuits, Helen's real-world experience comes from working with diverse individuals seeking personalized solutions for their health goals. Her compassionate and realistic approach to dieting resonates with those who value weight loss without sacrifice.

As a devoted wife, Helen recognizes the significance of family and shared meals. Her book reflects a deep understanding of the practical aspects of incorporating a low-carb lifestyle into a household, making it accessible for individuals and families alike.
Join Helen Munoz on a transformative journey through her Atkins Diet Book, where expertise, personal experience, and a genuine commitment to well-being converge to guide you toward a healthier, happier you.

Table of contents

INTRODUCTION

Step into the transformative realm of the Atkins Diet—a lifestyle that not only transforms our understanding of nutrition but also revolutionizes our approach to sustainable weight management. Built on the foundations of low-carbohydrate living, the Atkins Diet goes beyond traditional diet norms, guiding you on a voyage where gratifying meals and health-conscious choices intersect.

Embark on this culinary journey as we look into the four distinct phases of the Atkins Diet, each crafted to adapt to your evolving needs and aspirations. Get ready to relish tantalizing meals, revel in newfound energy, and witness the positive effects of controlled carbohydrate intake on your overall well-being. Whether you're a seasoned Atkins enthusiast or venturing onto this transformative path for the first time, this cookbook stands by you in creating flavorful, nutritious, and effortlessly enjoyable dishes. Embrace the Atkins lifestyle, where carb-conscious living meets culinary delight, and set forth on a journey towards a healthier, happier version of yourself.

Brief Overview Of The Atkins Diet

The Atkins diet is a low-carbohydrate diet that focuses on protein and fat consumption. Its goal is to get the body into a ketosis state, where it burns fat for energy. The diet is divided into four stages, beginning with a rigorous carbohydrate restriction and progressively reintroducing carbohydrates. According to research, critics worry about its long-term viability and associated health dangers, yet other individuals find it effective for short-term weight reduction.

Benefits Of Following The Atkins Diet

Concentrating on protein consumption and minimizing carbs, the Atkins diet stimulates the body to enter a state called ketosis. This metabolic state transfers the predominant energy source from glucose to stored fat, perhaps contributing to weight reduction. Additionally, reducing carb consumption will help regulate blood sugar levels, aiding patients with insulin resistance or diabetes.

The concentration of protein consumption in the Atkins diet adds to a sense of fullness, lowering total calorie intake. This, along with the metabolic benefits of ketosis, will result in more successful weight control.

Moreover, several researches i've done shows that the Atkins diet will favorably improve cardiovascular health. By lowering triglyceride levels and raising high-density lipoprotein (HDL) cholesterol, it will also contribute to a better lipid profile. However, long-term adherence and individual variances should be addressed when analyzing the diet's benefits to heart health.

In terms of energy levels, some persons on the Atkins diet report having improved vigor and decreased energy swings associated with carb-heavy diets. However, individual reactions to dietary modifications might differ, and it's crucial to monitor how the body reacts to such alterations.

BREAKFAST RECIPES

1. Atkins Low Carb Ham and Spinach Egg Bake

Net Carbs 8 grams
Prep Time: 15 Minutes
Method: American
Cooking Time: 22 Minutes
Difficulty level: Moderate
4 Servings

INGREDIENTS

- Original cooking spray
- 8 slices keto bread, Oroweat
- 1 cup frozen spinach, leaf, cut
- 5 lrgs raw egg
- 1/2 cup baked ham, cured, lean
- 3 tablespoons cottage cheese, 4% milk fat
- 2 tablespoons fresh scallions, tops & bulb, chopped
- 1/4 teaspoon table salt
- 1/4 teaspoon black pepper, ground

- 1/3 cup cheddar cheese, shredded

DIRECTIONS

Preheat your oven to 350°F (175°C) and apply cooking spray to eight muffin cups. Take keto bread slices, flatten them with a rolling pin, and cut each into four pieces. Arrange the bread quarters, slightly overlapping, around the edges of each muffin cup, placing the crust side down.

In a microwave-safe bowl, heat frozen spinach on high for two minutes. Squeeze excess liquid from the spinach using a clean kitchen or paper towel. Return spinach to the bowl, add eggs, diced ham, cottage cheese, chopped scallions, salt, and pepper. Mix thoroughly with a fork until ingredients are evenly distributed, ensuring no spinach lumps.

Distribute the egg mixture evenly among the prepared muffin cups, filling each with around two tablespoons of the mixture.

Sprinkle shredded cheddar cheese evenly over the top of each muffin cup.

Bake for 20 minutes or until the egg is fully cooked, and the bread edges begin to brown. Serve warm. Each serving comprises two egg bake cups. Store any leftovers in an airtight container in the refrigerator for up to four to five days and reheat in the microwave when needed.

---

2. Mexican Breakfast Pizza Recipe

Net Carbs 8.7 grams
Prep Time: 15 Minutes
Style:Mexican
Cook Time: 13 Minutes
Difficulty: Easy
4 Servings

INGREDIENTS

- 4 eas Carb Balance whole wheat tortilla, fajita, 6"

- 1 cup red salsa
- 4 lrgs raw egg
- 1/8 teaspoon table salt
- 1/8 teaspoon black pepper, ground
- 3/4 cup mexican blend cheese
- 1/2 ea fresh avocado
- 1 ea fresh jalapeno peppers
- 1 ounce queso fresco cheese
- 1/4 cup fresh radishes, sliced
- 2 eas fresh cilantro, sprig

DIRECTIONS

Preheat the oven to 350°F with the oven rack positioned in the top quarter. Place four tortillas on two parchment paper-lined sheet pans, ensuring even spacing. On each tortilla, add ¼ cup salsa in the center, forming a ring of salsa not quite reaching the tortilla's edge. Create a well in the middle of the salsa and gently crack an egg into it. Season with a pinch of salt and pepper, then sprinkle 3 tablespoons shredded cheese over the salsa.

Bake for 11-13 minutes until the egg whites are becoming opaque along the bottom. Switch the oven to broil for 2-3 minutes until the tops are opaque, and the yolk is cooked to your preference. Remove from the oven.

Top each tortilla pizza with about 25g of avocado, approximately 3g of sliced jalapeno, ¼ ounce crumbled queso fresco, around 8g of radish slices, and roughly chopped cilantro. Enjoy while warm. One pizza, as described above, constitutes one serving.

---

3. Strawberry Shortcake Bar Breakfast Bowl Recipe

Net Carbs 8.4 grams
Prep Time: 135 Minutes
Style: American
Cook Time: 0 Minutes
Difficulty: Easy
4 Servings

INGREDIENTS

- 1/4 cup Chia Seeds
- 1/4 cup Hemp Hearts
- 1 1/2 tablespoon(s) truvia sweet complete (2 tbsp= 21g)
- 1/2 tsp Cinnamon, ground
- 1 1/2 cup Almond Milk, plain, unsweetened
- 1 tsp Vanilla extract
- 1 cup Strawberries, fresh, sliced
- 1 1/3 cup Greek Yogurt, plain, unsweetened, whole milk
- 2 bar Atkins Strawberry Shortcake Bar

DIRECTIONS

Combine chia seeds, hemp hearts, 1 tablespoon sweetener, and cinnamon in a 16-ounce jar. Pour almond milk and vanilla, mix thoroughly, cover, and refrigerate for a minimum of 2 hours. Give it a shake or stir after approximately 1 hour.

In a small bowl, gently mix sliced strawberries with ½ tablespoon sweetener. Refrigerate for at least 10 minutes.

For assembly, place ¼ cup sliced strawberries on one side of each of 4 small bowls. Add 1/3 cup Greek yogurt and 1/3 cup of the chia pudding. Chop the bars and top each bowl with ½ bar.

---

4. Low Carb Healthy Acai Bowl

Net Carbs 11.5 grams
Prep Time: 20 Minutes
Style:American
Cook Time: 0 Minutes
Difficulty: Easy
1 Serving

INGREDIENTS

- 1 svg frozen acai smoothie mix, unsweetened
- 1/4 cup frozen blueberries, unsweetened

- 1 tablespoon allulose, liquid sweetener
- 1 tablespoon chia seeds
- 1 tablespoon almond butter
- 1 tablespoon coconut, shredded, unsweetened
- 5 eas fresh raspberries
- 1 tablespoon Hemp Hearts hemp seeds, shelled
- 1/2 bar Atkins Blueberry Soft Baked Energy Bar

DIRECTIONS

In a food processor, let frozen acai and frozen blueberries thaw at room temperature for approximately 15 minutes. Combine ¼ cup water and chia seeds in a small cup, letting it sit and stirring once or twice while the acai and blueberries thaw. Place the thawed acai and blueberries in a food processor, along with 2 teaspoons of hemp seeds and half of the almond butter. Process until smooth and transfer to a 12-ounce bowl.

Drizzle the remaining room temperature almond butter over the acai. Top with diced Atkins Blueberry Soft Baked Energy Bar, coconut shreds, raspberries, and the remaining 1 teaspoon of hemp seeds.

---

5. Cinnamon Buns

Net Carbs 4 grams
Prep Time: 80 Minutes
Style:American
Cook Time: 25 Minutes
Difficulty: Difficult
9 Servings

INGREDIENTS

- 2 tablespoons Tap Water
- 2 servings
- 2 tablespoons Cream, heavy, liquid
- 4 teaspoons butter, unsalted
- 2 tablespoons Inulin powder
- 1 pack Active Dry Yeast
- 1/4 cup Allulose, granulated

- 1 1/2 teaspoons Baking powder, double-acting, sodium aluminum
- 1 teaspoon Salt
- 2 each Egg (1 large fresh, whole, raw egg = 50g)
- 2 teaspoons Apple Cider Vinegar
- 1 tablespoon Whole Wheat Pastry Flour
- 2 2/3 tablespoons butter, unsalted
- 4 teaspoons Allulose, granulated
- 1 teaspoon Cinnamon, ground
- 6 tablespoons chopped pecans
- 1 ounce Currants, dried

DIRECTIONS

For this recipe, you'll need 2 cups (226 grams) of the Atkins Soy-Free Flour Mix. Keep in mind that one serving of the flour mix equals one cup, so 2 cups equate to 2 servings.

Prepare an 8-inch by 8-inch baking pan with parchment paper. In a small microwave-safe bowl, mix water, 4 teaspoons butter, cream, and inulin, then microwave for around 30 seconds on high. Stir until the butter melts and the inulin dissolves. The mixture's temperature should be about 110°F. Sprinkle yeast on top, cover with a kitchen towel, and let it rest in a warm spot for 7 minutes.

In a large bowl, combine flour mix, ¼ cup allulose, baking powder, and salt. Add room temperature eggs, apple cider vinegar, and the yeast mixture, folding together until a dough forms. Sprinkle some whole wheat flour on parchment paper, place the dough on top, and knead for about 4 minutes until it's less sticky. Set aside while you prepare the filling and warm the oven.

Preheat the oven to 150°F or the lowest setting possible. Once heated, turn the oven off. Melt 2 tablespoons and 2 teaspoons butter. Mix in 4 teaspoons allulose and cinnamon to create a paste.

Roll the dough into a 9-inch by 12-inch rectangle (about ¼-inch thick) using plastic wrap and parchment paper. Leave the lower 1-inch without filling, spread cinnamon butter evenly, then sprinkle chopped pecans and currants. Roll the dough into a tight log, cut into 9 rolls, and place them in the prepared baking pan.

Put the pan in the warm oven, leaving the door slightly open with a wooden spoon. Let the rolls rise for 1 hour. Remove from the oven, heat it to 350°F, and bake the rolls for 20-25 minutes until the tops are nicely browned. Serve warm, with one bun per serving.

---

6. Easy Low Carb Caramel French Toast Muffins

Net Carbs 3.9 grams
Prep Time: 15 Minutes
Style:American

Cook Time: 15 Minutes
Difficulty: Easy
8 Servings

INGREDIENTS

- 8 sec sprays canola oil cooking spray, non-aerosol
- 4 fl-oz Atkins Creamy Caramel Energy Shake
- 4 lrgs raw egg
- 1 teaspoon vanilla extract
- 1/8 teaspoon table salt
- 8 slices keto bread, Oroweat
- 1/4 cup pecans, chopped
- 1/4 cup caramel syrup, sugar free
- 1/2 cup heavy whipping cream

DIRECTIONS

Preheat the oven to 350°F and spray 8 wells of a muffin pan with oil. In a large bowl, whisk together Atkins Creamy Caramel Shake, eggs, vanilla, and salt until thoroughly mixed. Cut the bread into large cubes, add them to the bowl with eggs, and gently fold until all bread pieces are well coated in the egg mixture. Allow it to sit until the egg mixture is absorbed, around 5 minutes.

Evenly distribute the egg-soaked bread into the oiled wells of the muffin pan, ensuring each cup has 1 full piece of bread. Top each with ½ tablespoon of chopped pecans. Bake for 15 minutes or until set and fully cooked. Pour 1 teaspoon of sugar-free caramel syrup over each muffin and let them cool for 10 minutes.

While the muffins are cooling, use an electric mixer in a medium flat-bottom bowl to whip the heavy cream to soft peaks. Add the remaining 4 teaspoons of sugar-free caramel syrup and continue whipping to stiff peaks. Top each muffin with whipped cream, approximately 1 rounded tablespoon on each, and serve. One muffin, as described, constitutes one serving.

7. Low Carb Strawberry Almond Butter Porridge Recipe

Net Carbs 9.6 grams
Prep Time: 15 Minutes
Style:American
Cook Time: 10 Minutes
Difficulty: Easy
1 Serving

INGREDIENTS

- 1 cup coconut milk, enriched, unsweetened
- 1 tablespoon almond butter
- 1 teaspoon breakfast syrup, sugar free
- 3 tablespoons hemp seeds, hulled
- 2 tablespoons chia seeds
- 1 teaspoon butter, salted
- 4 lrgs fresh strawberries
- 1/2 bar Atkins Chocolate Almond Butter Bar

DIRECTIONS

Heat coconut milk in a small saucepan over medium heat until steaming. Stir in almond butter and sugar-free syrup until thoroughly blended.

In a cereal bowl, mix hemp and chia. Pour the warm milk mixture over and stir to combine, breaking up any clumps of chia seeds. Set aside while completing the recipe, stirring occasionally.

In a small non-stick skillet over medium heat, melt butter. Sauté sliced strawberries until warmed through and wilting, approximately 5 minutes. Place them on top of the porridge, along with chopped Atkins Chocolate Almond Butter bar, and serve while warm.

8. Bacon Shell Breakfast Tacos

Net Carbs 2.1 grams
Prep Time: 15 Minutes
Style:American
Cook Time: 25 Minutes
Difficulty: Moderate
6 Servings

INGREDIENTS

- 18 slices raw bacon, cured
- 1/4 teaspoon powder chili peppers
- 4 lrgs raw egg
- 1 tablespoon heavy whipping cream
- 1/4 teaspoon table salt
- 1 tablespoon butter, unsalted
- 1 1/2 tablespoons fresh scallions, tops & bulb, chopped
- 2 tablespoons mexican blend cheese
- 2 tablespoons red salsa
- 3/4 teaspoon fresh chives
- 1/2 tablespoon fresh cilantro, leaves
- 1/2 ea fresh avocado

DIRECTIONS

Preheat the oven to 400°F and line a baking sheet with foil. To create woven bacon taco shells, cut two bacon slices in half, then slice each half lengthwise to yield four skinny bacon strips. Weave these tightly, then take one more bacon piece, cut in half, and weave around the edges to form a round shape. Repeat until you have 6 round bacon mat shells. Sprinkle each with a pinch of chili powder. Cover with parchment paper and another baking sheet to keep the bacon flat. Bake for 20-25 minutes until fully cooked and starting to crisp. Shape into taco shells between two mugs while still warm and let cool completely.

In a medium bowl, whisk together eggs, salt, and heavy cream with a fork. Warm a skillet over medium heat, add butter, and sauté sliced scallions until just beginning to soften (about 1 minute). Add eggs and cook, stirring gently with a spatula until they reach the desired doneness, approximately 4 minutes more.

Evenly fill bacon shells with scrambled eggs, about 2 rounded tablespoons in each. Top each with 1 teaspoon shredded cheese, 1 teaspoon salsa, 1/8 teaspoon chopped fresh chives, 2 cilantro leaves, and an equal amount of avocado (around 11 grams each). One filled bacon shell, as described, constitutes one serving.

---

9. Low Carb Cinnamon Protein Porridge

Net Carbs 6.6 grams
Prep Time: 5 Minutes
Style:American
Cook Time: 5 Minutes
Difficulty: Easy
1 Serving

INGREDIENTS

- 1/4 cup flaxseed meal
- 2 tablespoons chia seeds
- 1/2 teaspoon cinnamon, ground
- 1 pinch table salt
- 6 fl-oz Atkins Creamy Cinnamon Swirl Shake
- 10 eas fresh blueberries
- 10 eas pecans, halves
- 1 tablespoon sugar free maple flavor syrup, Maple Grove Farms

DIRECTIONS

Ingredient tip: For optimal results, use a coffee grinder to grind flax seeds into fresh flaxseed meal for this recipe.

In a heat-resistant cereal bowl, mix together flaxseed meal, chia seeds, cinnamon, and salt. In a small saucepan over medium heat, warm Atkins Creamy Cinnamon Swirl Shake until steaming (about 5 minutes). Pour it into the bowl with the flaxseed meal mixture and stir until well combined. Allow it to sit for around 5 minutes, stirring occasionally, until it thickens. Top with blueberries, pecans, and sugar-free syrup. One bowl, as described, constitutes one serving.

---

10. Chai Latte Overnight Oats

Net Carbs 6.7 grams
Prep Time: 245 Minutes
Style:American
Cook Time: 3 Minutes
Difficulty: Easy
2 Servings

INGREDIENTS

- 2 tablespoon(s) Oats, quick cooking, raw (1 tbsp= 6 g)
- 2 tablespoons Hemp Hearts
- 2 tablespoons Chia Seeds
- 2 tablespoons Coconut, unsweetened, shredded

- 1 shake Atkins Chai Tea Latte Protein Shake
- 1 tablespoon Pine Nuts, roasted
- 1 teaspoon Coconut, unsweetened, shredded
- 1/16 teaspoon Cinnamon, ground

DIRECTIONS

In each of two 6-ounce jars with lids, combine 1 tablespoon oats, 1 tablespoon chia seeds, 1 tablespoon hemp hearts, and 1 tablespoon coconut shreds until evenly mixed. Pour half of the shake (5.5 fluid ounces) into each jar and thoroughly blend. Cover with lids and refrigerate for at least 4 hours or overnight.

Before serving, lightly toast pine nuts in a 400-degree oven for 3 minutes, shaking once halfway through. Garnish each jar with ½ tablespoon of roasted pine nuts, ½ teaspoon coconut shreds, and a pinch of cinnamon.

11. Cinnamon French Toast Recipe

Net Carbs 4 grams
Prep Time: 20 Minutes
Style:American
Cook Time: 20 Minutes
Difficulty: Moderate
6 Servings

INGREDIENTS

- 4 lrgs raw egg
- 4 fl-oz Atkins Creamy Cinnamon Swirl Shake
- 1 1/2 teaspoons vanilla extract
- 1/2 teaspoon cinnamon, ground
- 1 pinch table salt
- 6 slices keto bread, Oroweat
- 1 tablespoon butter, unsalted
- 6 tablespoons heavy whipping cream
- 2 tablespoons mascarpone cheese
- 1 tablespoon breakfast syrup, sugar free

DIRECTIONS

Whisk together eggs, Atkins Creamy Cinnamon Swirl Shake, 1 teaspoon vanilla extract, and cinnamon in a medium bowl. Pour into the bottom of a 9-inch by 13-inch baking pan, and place a single layer of bread on top. Let it soak for 5 minutes, flip, and allow another 5 minutes until the egg mixture is absorbed.

In a large skillet over medium-low heat, melt butter. Add a single layer of soaked bread and cook until browned (3-5 minutes). Flip, increase heat to medium, and cook until golden. Place on a plate in a warm oven (if needed) and repeat in batches for the remaining pieces of bread.

While the French toast is cooking, use a hand mixer on medium-high in a medium mixing bowl to whip together heavy cream and mascarpone until soft peaks form. Add sugar-free maple syrup and ½ teaspoon vanilla extract, mixing on medium until incorporated.

To serve, top each piece of French toast with a rounded 1/8 cup of whipped mascarpone. One piece of French toast with a rounded 1/8 cup of whipped mascarpone is one serving.

---

12. Low Carb Slow Cooker French Toast Casserole

Net Carbs 5.4 grams
Prep Time: 205 Minutes
Style:American
Cook Time: 150 Minutes
Difficulty: Easy
6 Servings

INGREDIENTS

- 4 buns of unbun buns
- 5 lrgs raw egg
- 1/2 cup heavy whipping cream

- 1/2 cup breakfast syrup, sugar free
- 2 teaspoons vanilla extract
- 2 1/2 teaspoons cinnamon, ground
- 1 teaspoon ginger, ground
- 1/4 teaspoon table salt
- 1/8 teaspoon nutmeg, ground
- 1/4 cup pecans, chopped
- 2 tablespoons Swerve sweetener, brown
- 2 tablespoons butter, unsalted

DIRECTIONS

Preheat the oven to 250°F and lightly grease a 6-quart slow cooker insert. Cube the bread and arrange it in a single layer on baking sheets. Toast in the oven for 20 minutes or until the bread cubes are dried out and crispy. Transfer them to the slow cooker.

In a blender, blend eggs, heavy cream, sugar-free maple syrup, vanilla, 2 teaspoons cinnamon, ginger, nutmeg, and 1/8 teaspoon salt. Pour this mixture over the bread cubes, pressing down to ensure thorough soaking. Refrigerate for at least 3 hours, ideally overnight, allowing the liquid to be absorbed into the bread cubes.

Remove the slow cooker insert from the refrigerator and let it come to room temperature for 30 minutes to 1 hour. In a small bowl, combine chopped pecans, brown Swerve, room temperature butter, ½ teaspoon cinnamon, and 1/8 teaspoon salt. Crumble this mixture evenly over the top of the casserole.
Cook in the slow cooker on high for 2-2 ½ hours or 4-4 ½ hours on low. The casserole is done when it no longer jiggles, and the temperature in the center of the casserole reaches 160°F.

---

13. Keto Migas with Nacho Protein Chips

Net Carbs 7 grams
Prep Time: 5 Minutes
Style:Mexican

Cook Time: 10 Minutes
Difficulty: Easy
2 Servings

INGREDIENTS

- 1/2 tablespoon canola oil
- 1/4 cup fresh green bell pepper, chopped
- 3 tablespoons fresh yellow onion, chopped
- 3 eas turkey breakfast sausage link
- 3 lrgs raw egg
- 1/4 teaspoon table salt
- 1 bag Atkins Nacho Cheese Protein Chips
- 1 ounce queso fresco cheese
- 2 tablespoons red salsa
- 1/2 ea fresh avocado
- 1 tablespoon sour cream
- 1 tablespoon fresh cilantro, leaves

DIRECTIONS

Heat canola oil in a medium non-stick skillet over medium heat. Add bell peppers, onions, and chopped precooked sausage, and sauté until onions are translucent, around 3-4 minutes.

In a small bowl, whisk together eggs and salt using a fork. Pour the eggs into the skillet with the vegetables and start scrambling. Add half the bag of chips and fold the egg mixture together until the eggs are fully scrambled, approximately 2 minutes more.

Remove from heat and fold in the remaining chips. Top with crumbled queso fresco, salsa, sliced avocado, sour cream, and cilantro. Serve immediately.

---

14. Italian Sausage Morning Soup

Net Carbs 8 grams
Prep Time: 10 Minutes
Style:Italian
Cook Time: 40 Minutes
Difficulty: Difficult
4 Servings

INGREDIENTS

1 tablespoon Extra Virgin Olive Oil
1/2 cup chopped Onions
1 stalk, medium (7-1/2" - 8" long) Celery
1/2 cup chopped Carrots
4 cups Chicken Broth, Bouillon or Consomme
1/4 cup Spaghetti/Marinara Pasta Sauce
1/4 teaspoon Italian Seasoning
8 ounces Italian Sausage, sweet
4 ounces Ground Beef (80% Lean / 20% Fat)
1 large Egg (Whole)

DIRECTIONS

In a large saucepan over medium heat, heat olive oil. Add white onion, diced celery, and carrots, and cook until they start to soften, approximately 5 minutes.

Add broth, marinara sauce, and Italian seasoning. Let it simmer for 20 minutes. Meanwhile, combine sausage, ground beef, and egg in a mixing bowl. Use a tablespoon to shape the meat mixture into balls and drop them into the simmering soup. Alternatively, you can bake the meatballs in a 350°F oven on a jelly roll pan until browned on the outside before adding them to the soup.

Continue cooking for an additional 20 minutes until the meatballs are thoroughly cooked. Season to taste with salt and freshly ground pepper, then serve immediately.

---

15. Low Carb Eggs and Spinach

Net Carbs 1.4 grams
Prep Time: 5 Minutes
Style:American
Cook Time: 5 Minutes
Difficulty: Moderate
1 Serving

INGREDIENTS

- 1 tablespoon Extra Virgin Olive Oil
- 2 cups Baby Spinach
- 2 large Eggs (Whole)

DIRECTIONS

Add oil to a small skillet over medium heat.

Add spinach and sauté until wilted.

Add eggs to skillet and scramble together until eggs are set.

Season to taste with salt and freshly ground black pepper before serving.

LUNCH RECIPES

1. Roast Beef, Red Bell Pepper and Provolone Lettuce Wraps Recipe

Net Carbs 2.7 grams
Prep Time: 5 Minutes
Style: American
Cook Time: 0 Minutes
Difficulty: Moderate
1 Serving

INGREDIENTS

- 2 inner leaves Romaine Lettuce (salad)
- 2 ounces Provolone Cheese
- 1 tablespoon Real Mayonnaise
- 1/2 teaspoon Horseradish
- 4 ounces boneless, cooked Roast Beef
- 1/4 medium (approx 2-3/4" long, 2-1/2" diameter) Red Sweet Pepper

DIRECTIONS

Take off the bottom part of lettuce leaves and place them flat on a clean surface. Add a slice of cheese on each leaf.

Mix mayonnaise with horseradish, and if desired, add garlic powder to taste. Season with salt and freshly ground black pepper. Spread this mixture onto the cheese slices, then layer with roast beef.

Slice the red bell pepper into 1/4-inch thick strips and arrange them on one end of the roast beef, cheese, and lettuce. Roll up the assembly, starting where the pepper strips are placed, until fully rolled. Secure with a toothpick, repeat for a second roll-up, and enjoy immediately.

2. Bacon-Egg Salad Flatout Wrap Recipe

Net Carbs 8.6 grams
Prep Time: 10 Minutes
Style:American
Cook Time: 0 Minutes
Difficulty: Moderate
1 Serving

INGREDIENTS

- 2 large Boiled Eggs
- 1 tablespoon Real Mayonnaise
- 1/2 tsp or 1 packet Yellow Mustard
- 1 flatbread Light Original Flatbread
- 1 1/2 oz, cooked Turkey Bacon
- 1 inner leaf Romaine Lettuce (salad)

DIRECTIONS

Mix together chopped eggs, mayonnaise and mustard. Add salt and pepper to taste.

Spread mixture on one rounded end of Flatout that has the lettuce flattened out on it. Top with cooked crumbled bacon then roll up and cut in half.

---

3. Zucchini Noodles with Pesto

Net Carbs: 7 grams
Prep Time: 20 minutes
Style: Vegetarian
Cook Time: 10 minutes
Difficulty: Moderate
No. Of Servings: 2

INGREDIENTS:

- 2 large zucchinis, spiralized
- 1 cup cherry tomatoes, halved
- 1/2 cup pesto sauce
- Pine nuts (optional)

INSTRUCTIONS:

Spiralize zucchini into noodle-like strands.
Sauté zucchini noodles until tender.
Toss with cherry tomatoes and pesto sauce.
Garnish with pine nuts if desired.

4. Turkey and Avocado Lettuce Wraps

Net Carbs: 4 grams
Prep Time: 10 minutes
Style: Quick and Easy
Cook Time: 0 minutes
Difficulty: Easy
No. Of Servings: 3

INGREDIENTS:
- 1 pound turkey slices
- 1 large avocado, sliced
- Lettuce leaves (e.g., iceberg or butter lettuce)
- Mustard or mayonnaise (optional)

INSTRUCTIONS:
Lay out lettuce leaves.
Add turkey slices and avocado.
Drizzle with mustard or mayonnaise if desired.
Roll up and secure with toothpicks.

5. Cauliflower Fried Rice

Net Carbs: 8 grams
Prep Time: 15 minutes
Style: Asian-Inspired
Cook Time: 15 minutes
Difficulty: Moderate
No. Of Servings: 4

INGREDIENTS:

- 1 medium cauliflower, grated
- 1 cup mixed vegetables (peas, carrots, corn)
- 2 eggs, beaten
- Soy sauce (low-carb)

INSTRUCTIONS:

Grate cauliflower to resemble rice.
Sauté mixed vegetables in a pan.
Push vegetables to the side, pour beaten eggs into the pan, and scramble.
Mix cauliflower rice into the pan and add soy sauce to taste.

6. Salmon Avocado Lettuce Wraps

Net Carbs: 3 grams
Prep Time: 20 minutes
Style: Seafood
Cook Time: 10 minutes
Difficulty: Moderate
No. Of Servings: 2

INGREDIENTS:

- 2 salmon filets
- 1 ripe avocado, sliced
- Lettuce leaves
- Lemon wedges for garnish

INSTRUCTIONS:

Grill or bake salmon filets until cooked.
Place salmon on lettuce leaves.
Top with sliced avocado.
Squeeze lemon juice over the top for extra flavor.

---

7. Egg Salad Stuffed Bell Peppers

Net Carbs: 6 grams
Prep Time: 15 minutes
Style: Quick and Easy
Cook Time: 0 minutes
Difficulty: Easy
No. Of Servings: 4

INGREDIENTS:

- 6 hard-boiled eggs, chopped
- 1/4 cup mayonnaise
- 1 celery stalk, finely chopped
- Bell peppers (various colors)

INSTRUCTIONS:

Mix chopped eggs, mayonnaise, and celery in a bowl.
Cut bell peppers in half and remove seeds.
Stuff each half with the egg salad mixture.

8. Shrimp and Broccoli Stir-Fry

Net Carbs: 5 grams
Prep Time: 20 minutes
Style: Stir-Fry
Cook Time: 15 minutes
Difficulty: Moderate
No. Of Servings: 3

INGREDIENTS:
- 1 pound shrimp, peeled and deveined
- 2 cups broccoli florets
- 1 bell pepper, sliced
- 2 tablespoons soy sauce (low-carb)

INSTRUCTIONS:
Stir-fry shrimp in a pan until pink and cooked.
Add broccoli and bell pepper to the pan.
Drizzle with low-carb soy sauce and toss until vegetables are tender.

9. Beef and Vegetable Skewers

Net Carbs: 6 grams
Prep Time: 25 minutes
Style: BBQ
Cook Time: 15 minutes
Difficulty: Moderate
No. Of Servings: 4

INGREDIENTS:
- 1 pound beef sirloin, cut into cubes
- Bell peppers, onions, and cherry tomatoes for skewering
- Low-carb BBQ sauce

INSTRUCTIONS:
Thread beef cubes and vegetables onto skewers.

Grill skewers until beef is cooked to your liking.

Brush with low-carb BBQ sauce during grilling.

10. Spinach and Feta Stuffed Chicken Breast

Net Carbs: 3 grams
Prep Time: 20 minutes
Style: Mediterranean
Cook Time: 25 minutes
Difficulty: Moderate
No. Of Servings: 2

INGREDIENTS:
- 2 boneless, skinless chicken breasts
- 1 cup fresh spinach, chopped
- Feta cheese, crumbled
- Olive oil

INSTRUCTIONS:
Preheat the oven to 375°F (190°C).
Butterfly chicken breasts and stuff with spinach and feta.
Secure with toothpicks and bake until chicken is cooked through.

11. Turkey and Cheese Lettuce Wraps

Net Carbs: 2 grams
Prep Time: 10 minutes
Style: Quick and Easy
Cook Time: 0 minutes
Difficulty: Easy
No. Of Servings: 3

INGREDIENTS:
- Turkey slices
- Cheese slices (e.g., cheddar or Swiss)
- Lettuce leaves

INSTRUCTIONS:
Layer turkey and cheese on lettuce leaves.
Roll up and secure with toothpicks.

12. Cucumber and Smoked Salmon Bites

Net Carbs: 2 grams
Prep Time: 15 minutes
Style: Seafood
Cook Time: 0 minutes
Difficulty: Easy
No. Of Servings: 4

INGREDIENTS:

- Cucumber, sliced
- Smoked salmon
- Cream cheese (full-fat)

INSTRUCTIONS:

Top cucumber slices with a small dollop of cream cheese.
Add a piece of smoked salmon on top.

13. Avocado and Bacon Egg Salad

Net Carbs: 4 grams
Prep Time: 15 minutes
Style: Quick and Easy
Cook Time: 10 minutes
Difficulty: Easy
No. Of Servings: 2

INGREDIENTS:

- 4 hard-boiled eggs, chopped
- 1 avocado, diced
- Cooked bacon, crumbled
- Mayonnaise

INSTRUCTIONS:

Combine chopped eggs, diced avocado, and crumbled bacon in a bowl.
Mix in mayonnaise to desired consistency.

14. Chicken and Vegetable Casserole

Net Carbs: 8 grams
Prep Time: 30 minutes
Style: Casserole
Cook Time: 25 minutes
Difficulty:Moderate
No. Of Servings: 6

INGREDIENTS:

- 2 cups cooked chicken, shredded
- Mixed vegetables (broccoli, cauliflower, bell peppers)
- Cream cheese (full-fat)
- Shredded cheddar cheese

INSTRUCTIONS:

Preheat the oven to 375°F (190°C).
Mix shredded chicken and vegetables in a baking dish.
Blend in cream cheese and top with shredded cheddar.

Bake until the cheese is melted and bubbly.

---

15. Tuna Salad Stuffed Avocados

Net Carbs: 6 grams
Prep Time: 15 minutes
Style: Seafood
Cook Time: 0 minutes
Difficulty: Easy
No. Of Servings: 4

INGREDIENTS:
- 2 cans tuna, drained
- Celery, finely chopped
- Red onion, finely chopped
- Mayonnaise

INSTRUCTIONS:
In a bowl, mix tuna, chopped celery, red onion, and mayonnaise.
Cut avocados in half and remove pits.
Spoon tuna salad into avocado halves.

DINNER RECIPES

1. Lemon Garlic Butter Shrimp

Net Carbs: 3 grams
Prep Time: 15 minutes
Style: Sauteed
Cook Time: 5 minutes
Difficulty: Easy
No. Of SERVINGS: 4

INGREDIENTS:
- 1 lb shrimp (peeled and deveined)
- 3 tablespoons butter
- 4 cloves garlic (minced)
- Juice of 2 lemons
- Salt and pepper to taste
- Fresh parsley for garnish

DIRECTIONS:
In a skillet, melt butter over medium heat. Add minced garlic and sauté until fragrant. Add shrimp, cook for 2-3 minutes per side or until pink.

Squeeze lemon juice over shrimp, season with salt and pepper.
Garnish with fresh parsley before serving.

---

2. Cauliflower and Broccoli Cheese Bake

Net Carbs: 6 grams
Prep Time: 20 minutes
Style: Baked
Cook Time: 30 minutes
Difficulty: Moderate
No. Of SERVINGS: 6

INGREDIENTS:

- 1 head cauliflower (cut into florets)
- 2 cups broccoli florets
- 1 cup heavy cream
- 2 cups shredded cheddar cheese
- 1/2 cup grated Parmesan cheese
- 2 cloves garlic (minced)
- Salt and pepper to taste

DIRECTIONS:
Preheat the oven to 375°F (190°C).
Steam cauliflower and broccoli until slightly tender.
In a saucepan, heat heavy cream, garlic, and cheeses until melted.
Place steamed vegetables in a baking dish, pour cheese mixture over, and bake for 25-30 minutes.

---

3. Greek Salad with Grilled Chicken

Net Carbs: 8 grams
Prep Time: 25 minutes
Style: Grilled
Cook Time: 15 minutes
Difficulty: Easy
No. Of SERVINGS: 4

INGREDIENTS:
- 1.5 lbs chicken breast (thinly sliced)
- 1 cucumber (diced)
- 1 cup cherry tomatoes (halved)

- 1/2 cup Kalamata olives (sliced)
- 1/2 cup feta cheese (crumbled)
- 1/4 cup red onion (thinly sliced)
- 2 tablespoons olive oil
- Juice of 1 lemon
- 1 teaspoon dried oregano
- Salt and pepper to taste

DIRECTIONS:

Season chicken slices with oregano, salt, and pepper. Grill until cooked through.

In a bowl, combine cucumber, tomatoes, olives, feta, and red onion.

Drizzle olive oil and lemon juice over the salad, toss gently.

Top the salad with grilled chicken slices.

---

4. Spinach and Artichoke Stuffed Chicken

Net Carbs: 4 grams
Prep Time: 30 minutes
Style: Baked

Cook Time: 25 minutes
Difficulty: Moderate
No. Of SERVINGS: 4

INGREDIENTS:

- 4 boneless, skinless chicken breasts
- 1 cup fresh spinach (chopped)
- 1 cup artichoke hearts (chopped)
- 1/2 cup cream cheese
- 1/4 cup grated Parmesan cheese
- 2 cloves garlic (minced)
- Salt and pepper to taste

DIRECTIONS:

Preheat the oven to 375°F (190°C).

In a bowl, mix spinach, artichokes, cream cheese, Parmesan, and minced garlic.

Cut a pocket into each chicken breast, stuff with the mixture, and secure with toothpicks.

Season chicken with salt and pepper, then bake for 25 minutes.

5. Eggplant Parmesan

Net Carbs: 9 grams
Prep Time: 40 minutes
Style: Baked
Cook Time: 30 minutes
Difficulty: Moderate
No. Of SERVINGS: 6

INGREDIENTS:

- 2 large eggplants (sliced)
- 2 cups marinara sauce (sugar-free)
- 2 cups shredded mozzarella cheese
- 1 cup grated Parmesan cheese
- 1 cup almond flour
- 2 eggs (beaten)
- 2 teaspoons dried basil
- 1 teaspoon garlic powder
- Salt and pepper to taste

DIRECTIONS:

Preheat the oven to 375°F (190°C).

Mix almond flour, dried basil, garlic powder, salt, and pepper.

Dip eggplant slices in beaten eggs, then coat with the almond flour mixture.

Bake coated slices for 15 minutes. In a baking dish, layer eggplant, marinara sauce, and cheeses. Repeat.

Bake for an additional 20-25 minutes until bubbly and golden.

---

6. Cilantro Lime Chicken Thighs

Net Carbs:1 gram
Prep Time: 25 minutes
Style: Grilled
Cook Time: 20 minutes
Difficulty: Easy
No. Of SERVINGS: 4

INGREDIENTS:
- 8 bone-in, skin-on chicken thighs
- 1/4 cup fresh cilantro (chopped)
- 2 limes (juiced)

- 2 tablespoons olive oil
- 2 teaspoons ground cumin
- 1 teaspoon paprika
- Salt and pepper to taste

DIRECTIONS:
Preheat the grill to medium-high heat.
In a bowl, mix chopped cilantro, lime juice, olive oil, cumin, paprika, salt, and pepper.
Rub the mixture over chicken thighs.
Grill chicken for 20 minutes, turning occasionally, until juices run clear.

---

7. Caprese Stuffed Avocado

Net Carbs: 7 grams
Prep Time: 15 minutes
Style: Fresh
Cook Time: 0 minutes
Difficulty: Easy
No. Of SERVINGS: 4

INGREDIENTS:

- 2 avocados (halved and pitted)
- 1 cup cherry tomatoes (halved)
- 1 cup fresh mozzarella balls (mini)
- 1/4 cup fresh basil leaves (chopped)
- 2 tablespoons balsamic glaze
- Salt and pepper to taste

DIRECTIONS:

Scoop out a bit of avocado from each half to create a well.

In a bowl, combine cherry tomatoes, mozzarella, basil, salt, and pepper.

Stuff avocado halves with the caprese mixture.

Drizzle balsamic glaze over the top and serve.

---

8. Buffalo Chicken Lettuce Wraps

Net Carbs: 3 grams
Prep Time: 20 minutes
Style: Fresh

Cook Time: 10 minutes
Difficulty: Easy
No. Of SERVINGS: 4

INGREDIENTS:

- 1 lb ground chicken
- 1/2 cup buffalo sauce
- 1/2 cup celery (diced)
- 1/4 cup blue cheese (crumbled)
- 1/4 cup ranch dressing
- 1 head iceberg lettuce (leaves separated)

DIRECTIONS:

In a skillet, cook ground chicken until browned.

Mix in buffalo sauce and diced celery.

Spoon the buffalo chicken mixture into lettuce leaves.

Top with blue cheese crumbles and a drizzle of ranch dressing.

---

9. Beef and Vegetable Stir-Fry

Net Carbs: 6 grams
Prep Time: 25 minutes
Style: Stir-Fry
Cook Time: 15 minutes
Difficulty: Moderate
No. Of SERVINGS: 4

INGREDIENTS:
- 1 lb beef sirloin (sliced thinly)
- 2 cups broccoli florets
- 1 bell pepper (sliced)
- 1 cup snap peas
- 3 tablespoons soy sauce (low-carb)
- 2 tablespoons sesame oil
- 2 cloves garlic (minced)
- 1 tablespoon ginger (grated)

DIRECTIONS:
Marinate sliced beef in soy sauce, minced garlic, and grated ginger for 20 minutes.

Heat sesame oil in a wok or skillet. Stir-fry beef until browned.

Add broccoli, bell pepper, and snap peas. Continue stir-frying until vegetables are crisp-tender.

---

10. Turkey and Spinach Stuffed Mushrooms

Net Carbs: 4 grams
Prep Time: 30 minutes
Style: Baked
Cook Time: 20 minutes
Difficulty: Moderate
No. Of SERVINGS: 6

INGREDIENTS:

- 24 large mushrooms (stems removed)
- 1 lb ground turkey
- 2 cups fresh spinach (chopped)
- 1/2 cup cream cheese
- 1/4 cup grated Parmesan cheese
- 2 cloves garlic (minced)

- Salt and pepper to taste

DIRECTIONS:
Preheat the oven to 375°F (190°C).
In a skillet, cook ground turkey until browned. Add chopped spinach and minced garlic, cook until wilted.
In a bowl, mix turkey mixture with cream cheese and Parmesan.
Stuff mushrooms with the turkey mixture and bake for 20 minutes.

---

11. Pesto Zoodle Bowl with Grilled Chicken

Net Carbs: 5 grams
Prep Time: 20 minutes
Style: Fresh
Cook Time: 10 minutes
Difficulty: Easy
No. Of SERVINGS: 4

INGREDIENTS:

- 4 zucchinis (spiralized)
- 1.5 lbs chicken breast (grilled and sliced)
- 1 cup cherry tomatoes (halved)
- 1/2 cup pine nuts (toasted)
- 1/2 cup basil pesto
- 2 tablespoons olive oil
- Salt and pepper to taste

DIRECTIONS:

In a pan, sauté zoodles in olive oil until just tender.

Toss grilled chicken, cherry tomatoes, and toasted pine nuts with the zoodles.

Drizzle basil pesto over the mixture, season with salt and pepper, and serve.

---

12. Shrimp and Avocado Salad

Net Carbs: 4 grams
Prep Time: 15 minutes
Style: Fresh

Cook Time: 0 minutes
Difficulty: Easy
No. Of SERVINGS: 2

INGREDIENTS:

- 1 lb shrimp (peeled and deveined)
- 2 avocados (diced)
- 1 cup cucumber (diced)
- 1/4 cup red onion (finely chopped)
- 2 tablespoons cilantro (chopped)
- Juice of 2 limes
- 1 tablespoon olive oil
- Salt and pepper to taste

DIRECTIONS:

Boil or sauté shrimp until cooked. Let them cool.

In a bowl, combine shrimp, diced avocados, cucumber, red onion, and cilantro.

Drizzle lime juice and olive oil over the salad, season with salt and pepper, and toss gently.

---

13. Low-Carb Meatball Casserole

Net Carbs: 5 grams
Prep Time: 30 minutes
Style: Baked
Cook Time: 25 minutes
Difficulty: Moderate
No. Of SERVINGS: 6

INGREDIENTS:

- 1.5 lbs ground beef
- 1 cup almond flour
- 1/2 cup grated Parmesan cheese
- 2 cloves garlic (minced)
- 2 teaspoons dried oregano
- 2 cups marinara sauce (sugar-free)
- 2 cups shredded mozzarella cheese
- Fresh basil for garnish
- Salt and pepper to taste

DIRECTIONS:
Preheat the oven to 375°F (190°C).
In a bowl, mix ground beef, almond flour, Parmesan, minced garlic, oregano, salt, and pepper. Form into meatballs.
Brown meatballs in a skillet. Place in a baking dish, cover with marinara sauce and mozzarella.
Bake for 25 minutes or until cheese is melted and bubbly. Garnish with fresh basil.

---

14. Avocado Lime Chicken Salad

Net Carbs: 6 grams
Prep Time: 20 minutes
Style: Fresh
Cook Time: 0 minutes
Difficulty: Easy
No. Of SERVINGS: 4

INGREDIENTS:

- 1.5 lbs chicken breast (cooked and shredded)
- 2 avocados (diced)
- 1 cup cherry tomatoes (halved)
- 1/4 cup red onion (finely chopped)
- 1/4 cup fresh cilantro (chopped)
- Juice of 3 limes
- 2 tablespoons olive oil
- Salt and pepper to taste

DIRECTIONS:

In a bowl, combine shredded chicken, diced avocados, cherry tomatoes, red onion, and cilantro.

Drizzle lime juice and olive oil over the salad. Season with salt and pepper, and toss gently.

15.　Broccoli　Cheddar　Stuffed Chicken

Net Carbs: 5 grams
Prep Time: 35 minutes
Style: Baked
Cook Time: 30 minutes
Difficulty: Moderate
No. Of SERVINGS: 4

INGREDIENTS:

- 4 boneless, skinless chicken breasts
- 2 cups broccoli florets (steamed)
- 1.5 cups shredded cheddar cheese
- 1/4 cup mayonnaise
- 2 tablespoons Dijon mustard
- 1 clove garlic (minced)
- Salt and pepper to taste

DIRECTIONS:

Preheat the oven to 375°F (190°C).
Cut a pocket into each chicken breast. In a bowl, mix steamed broccoli, cheddar,

mayonnaise, Dijon, minced garlic, salt, and pepper.
Stuff chicken breasts with the broccoli mixture. Bake for 30 minutes or until chicken is cooked through.

DESSERT RECIPES

1. Keto Chocolate Avocado Mousse

Net Carbs: 4g
Prep Time: 15 minutes
Style: Chilled
Cook Time: 0 minutes
Difficulty: Easy
No. Of SERVINGS: 4

INGREDIENTS:

- 2 ripe avocados
- 1/2 cup unsweetened cocoa powder
- 1/2 cup almond milk
- 1/4 cup powdered erythritol
- 1 teaspoon vanilla extract
- Pinch of salt
- Whipped cream for garnish

DIRECTIONS:

Blend avocados, cocoa powder, almond milk, erythritol, vanilla extract, and salt until smooth.

Chill in the refrigerator for at least 2 hours. Serve topped with whipped cream.

---

2. Berry Almond Chia Pudding

Net Carbs: 6g
Prep Time: 10 minutes
Style: Chilled
Cook Time: 0 minutes
Difficulty: Easy
No. Of SERVINGS: 2

INGREDIENTS:
- 1 cup unsweetened almond milk
- 1/4 cup chia seeds
- 1/2 cup mixed berries (strawberries, blueberries, raspberries)
- 1/4 cup sliced almonds
- 1 tablespoon powdered erythritol
- 1/2 teaspoon vanilla extract

DIRECTIONS:

Mix almond milk, chia seeds, erythritol, and vanilla extract in a bowl.

Let it sit in the refrigerator for at least 4 hours or overnight.

Before serving, layer chia pudding with mixed berries and sliced almonds.

---

3. Lemon Coconut Fat Bombs

Net Carbs: 1g
Prep Time: 15 minutes
Style: Chilled
Cook Time: 0 minutes
Difficulty: Easy
No. Of SERVINGS: 8

INGREDIENTS:
- 1/2 cup coconut oil (melted)
- 1/4 cup unsweetened shredded coconut
- 2 tablespoons lemon juice
- Zest of 1 lemon

- 2 tablespoons powdered erythritol

DIRECTIONS:
Mix melted coconut oil, shredded coconut, lemon juice, lemon zest, and erythritol.
Spoon into silicone molds or ice cube trays.
Freeze until solid, then pop out and enjoy.

---

4. Almond Butter Chocolate Cups

Net Carbs: 3g
Prep Time: 20 minutes
Style: Chilled
Cook Time: 0 minutes
Difficulty: Easy
No. Of SERVINGS: 6

INGREDIENTS:
- 1/2 cup almond butter
- 1/4 cup coconut oil (melted)
- 2 tablespoons unsweetened cocoa powder
- 2 tablespoons powdered erythritol

- Pinch of salt

DIRECTIONS:
Mix almond butter, melted coconut oil, cocoa powder, erythritol, and salt until smooth.
Spoon into silicone molds or mini cupcake liners.
Chill in the refrigerator until set.

---

5. Vanilla Cheesecake Bites

Net Carbs: 2g
Prep Time: 15 minutes
Style: Chilled
Cook Time: 0 minutes
Difficulty: Easy
No. Of SERVINGS: 8

INGREDIENTS:
- 1 cup cream cheese (softened)
- 1/4 cup powdered erythritol
- 1 teaspoon vanilla extract

- 1/4 cup heavy cream
- Berries for garnish

DIRECTIONS:
Beat cream cheese, erythritol, vanilla extract, and heavy cream until smooth.
Spoon into small serving cups.
Chill in the refrigerator for at least 2 hours.
Garnish with berries before serving.

---

6. Pumpkin Spice Fat Bombs

Net Carbs: 3g
Prep Time: 20 minutes
Style: Chilled
Cook Time: 0 minutes
Difficulty: Easy
No. Of SERVINGS: 12

- Ingredients:
- 1/2 cup pumpkin puree
- 1/4 cup coconut oil (melted)
- 2 tablespoons almond butter

- 2 tablespoons powdered erythritol
- 1 teaspoon pumpkin spice

DIRECTIONS:
Mix pumpkin puree, melted coconut oil, almond butter, erythritol, and pumpkin spice.
Spoon into silicone molds.
Freeze until solid, then enjoy.

---

7. Chocolate Almond Butter Cups

Net Carbs: 4g
Prep Time: 15 minutes
Style: Chilled
Cook Time: 0 minutes
Difficulty: Easy
No. Of SERVINGS: 8

INGREDIENTS:
- 1/2 cup almond butter
- 1/4 cup coconut oil (melted)

- 2 tablespoons unsweetened cocoa powder
- 2 tablespoons powdered erythritol
- 1/2 teaspoon vanilla extract
- Pinch of salt

DIRECTIONS:

Mix almond butter, melted coconut oil, cocoa powder, erythritol, vanilla extract, and salt until well combined.

Spoon the mixture into mini cupcake liners or silicone molds.

Chill in the refrigerator until set.

---

8. Cinnamon Pecan Keto Mug Cake

Net Carbs: 5g
Prep Time: 5 minutes
Style: Microwave
Cook Time: 2 minutes
Difficulty: Easy
No. Of SERVINGS: 1

INGREDIENTS:

- 3 tablespoons almond flour
- 1 tablespoon coconut flour
- 1 tablespoon powdered erythritol
- 1/4 teaspoon baking powder
- 1/4 teaspoon cinnamon
- 2 tablespoons pecans (chopped)
- 2 tablespoons unsweetened almond milk
- 1 tablespoon melted butter
- 1/4 teaspoon vanilla extract

DIRECTIONS:

In a mug, mix almond flour, coconut flour, erythritol, baking powder, cinnamon, and chopped pecans.

Add almond milk, melted butter, and vanilla extract. Stir until well combined.

Microwave for 2 minutes or until the cake is set.

---

9 Coconut Lime Fat Bombs

Net Carbs: 1g
Prep Time: 15 minutes
Style: Chilled
Cook Time: 0 minutes
Difficulty: Easy
No. Of SERVINGS: 10

INGREDIENTS:

- 1/2 cup coconut butter
- 1/4 cup coconut oil (melted)
- Zest of 2 limes
- 2 tablespoons powdered erythritol
- 1/2 teaspoon vanilla extract
- Unsweetened shredded coconut for coating

DIRECTIONS:

In a bowl, mix coconut butter, melted coconut oil, lime zest, erythritol, and vanilla extract.

Shape the mixture into small balls and roll in shredded coconut.
Freeze until firm, then serve.

---

10   Chocolate   Mint   Avocado Pudding

Net Carbs: 5g
Prep Time: 10 minutes
Style: Chilled
Cook Time: 0 minutes
Difficulty: Easy
No. Of SERVINGS: 4

INGREDIENTS:
2 ripe avocados
1/4 cup unsweetened cocoa powder
1/4 cup almond milk
1/4 cup powdered erythritol
1/2 teaspoon peppermint extract
Whipped cream for garnish

DIRECTIONS:

Blend avocados, cocoa powder, almond milk, erythritol, and peppermint extract until smooth.
Chill in the refrigerator for at least 1 hour.
Top with whipped cream before serving.

---

11 Almond Flour Lemon Poppy Seed Muffins

Net Carbs: 3g
Prep Time: 15 minutes
Style: Baked
Cook Time: 20 minutes
Difficulty: Easy
No. Of SERVINGS: 6

INGREDIENTS:

- 1 cup almond flour
- 2 tablespoons coconut flour
- 1/4 cup powdered erythritol
- 1/2 teaspoon baking powder
- Zest of 1 lemon

- 2 tablespoons poppy seeds
- 2 large eggs
- 1/4 cup unsweetened almond milk
- 2 tablespoons melted butter
- 1 teaspoon vanilla extract

DIRECTIONS:
Preheat the oven to 350°F (175°C). Line a muffin tin with paper liners.
In a bowl, mix almond flour, coconut flour, erythritol, baking powder, lemon zest, and poppy seeds.
In a separate bowl, whisk eggs, almond milk, melted butter, and vanilla extract.
Combine wet and dry ingredients. Spoon into muffin cups and bake for 20 minutes.

---

12. Raspberry Almond Chia Seed and Pudding

Net Carbs: 6g
Prep Time: 10 minutes
Style: Chilled

Cook Time: 0 minutes
Difficulty: Easy
No. Of SERVINGS: 2

INGREDIENTS:

- 1 cup unsweetened almond milk
- 1/4 cup chia seeds
- 1/2 cup fresh raspberries
- 2 tablespoons sliced almonds
- 1 tablespoon powdered erythritol
- 1/2 teaspoon vanilla extract

DIRECTIONS:

Mix almond milk, chia seeds, erythritol, and vanilla extract in a bowl.

Let it sit in the refrigerator for at least 4 hours or overnight.

Before serving, top with fresh raspberries and sliced almonds.

13. Chocolate Hazelnut Fat Bombs

Net Carbs: 2g
Prep Time: 15 minutes
Style: Chilled
Cook Time: 0 minutes
Difficulty: Easy
No. Of SERVINGS: 10

INGREDIENTS:

- 1/2 cup hazelnut butter
- 1/4 cup coconut oil (melted)
- 2 tablespoons unsweetened cocoa powder
- 2 tablespoons powdered erythritol
- 1/2 teaspoon vanilla extract
- Chopped hazelnuts for coating

DIRECTIONS:

Mix hazelnut butter, melted coconut oil, cocoa powder, erythritol, and vanilla extract. Shape the mixture into small balls and roll in chopped hazelnuts.

Freeze until firm, then enjoy.

---

14. Blueberry Almond Flour Mug Cake

Net Carbs: 4g
Prep Time: 5 minutes
Style: Microwave
Cook Time: 2 minutes
Difficulty: Easy
No. Of SERVINGS: 1

INGREDIENTS:
- 3 tablespoons almond flour
- 1 tablespoon coconut flour
- 1 tablespoon powdered erythritol
- 1/4 teaspoon baking powder
- 1/4 cup blueberries
- 2 tablespoons unsweetened almond milk
- 1 tablespoon melted butter
- 1/4 teaspoon almond extract

DIRECTIONS:

In a mug, mix almond flour, coconut flour, erythritol, baking powder, and blueberries. Add almond milk, melted butter, and almond extract. Stir until well combined. Microwave for 2 minutes or until the cake is set.

---

15. Coconut Flour Lemon Bars

Net Carbs: 5g
Prep Time: 20 minutes
Style: Baked
Cook Time: 25 minutes
Difficulty: Moderate
No. Of SERVINGS: 9

INGREDIENTS:

- 1 cup coconut flour
- 1/2 cup melted coconut oil
- 1/4 cup powdered erythritol
- Zest and juice of 2 lemons
- 4 large eggs

- 1/2 teaspoon vanilla extract

DIRECTIONS:

Heat the oven to 350°F (175°C) and grease a square baking pan. In a bowl, combine coconut flour, melted coconut oil, erythritol, lemon zest, and vanilla extract. Press the mixture into the bottom of the prepared pan.

Bake for 10 minutes. While baking, whisk together lemon juice and eggs. Pour the lemon mixture over the crust and bake for an additional 15 minutes.

Allow it to cool, then refrigerate before cutting into bars.

SNACK RECIPES

1. Cucumber and Cream Cheese Bites

Net Carbs: 2g
Prep Time: 10 minutes
Style: Fresh
Cook Time: 0 minutes
Difficulty: Easy
No. Of SERVINGS: 4

INGREDIENTS:
- 1 cucumber (sliced)
- 1/2 cup cream cheese
- Smoked salmon or deli turkey slices
- Fresh dill for garnish

DIRECTIONS:
Spread cream cheese on cucumber slices.
Top with smoked salmon or deli turkey.
Garnish with fresh dill and serve.

2. Spicy Roasted Almonds

Net Carbs: 3g
Prep Time: 15 minutes
Style: Roasted
Cook Time: 15 minutes
Difficulty: Easy
No. Of SERVINGS: 6

INGREDIENTS:
- 2 cups raw almonds
- 2 tablespoons olive oil
- 1 teaspoon paprika
- 1/2 teaspoon cayenne pepper
- 1 teaspoon garlic powder
- Add Salt to taste

DIRECTIONS:
Preheat the oven to 350°F (175°C).
Toss almonds with olive oil, paprika, cayenne pepper, and garlic powder.
Spread on a baking sheet and roast for 15 minutes, stirring halfway.

Sprinkle with salt while still warm.

---

3. Egg Salad Lettuce Wraps

Net Carbs: 2g
Prep Time: 15 minutes
Style: Fresh
Cook Time: 0 minutes
Difficulty: Easy
No. Of SERVINGS: 4

INGREDIENTS:

- 6 hard-boiled eggs (chopped)
- 1/4 cup mayonnaise
- 1 tablespoon Dijon mustard
- 2 tablespoons chives (chopped)
- Salt and pepper to taste
- Large lettuce leaves

DIRECTIONS:

In a bowl, mix chopped hard-boiled eggs, mayonnaise, Dijon mustard, chives, salt, and pepper.

Spoon the egg salad onto large lettuce leaves.
Roll the leaves to create lettuce wraps.

---

4. Zucchini Pizza Bites

Net Carbs: 4g
Prep Time: 20 minutes
Style: Baked
Cook Time: 15 minutes
Difficulty: Moderate
No. Of SERVINGS: 4

INGREDIENTS:
- 2 large zucchinis (sliced)
- 1/2 cup marinara sauce (sugar-free)
- 1 cup shredded mozzarella cheese
- 1/4 cup sliced pepperoni or your favorite toppings
- Italian seasoning

DIRECTIONS:

Preheat the oven to 400°F (200°C).

2. Place zucchini slices on a baking sheet.

3. Top with marinara sauce, mozzarella, and your chosen toppings.

4. Sprinkle it with Italian seasoning and bake for 15 minutes.

---

5. Bacon-Wrapped Jalapeño Poppers

Net Carbs: 1g

Prep Time: 20 minutes

Style: Baked

Cook Time: 15 minutes

Difficulty: Moderate

No. Of SERVINGS: 6

INGREDIENTS:

12 jalapeños (halved and seeded)

1 cup cream cheese

12 slices bacon

DIRECTIONS:

Preheat the oven to 400°F (200°C).

Fill each jalapeño half with cream cheese.

Wrap each jalapeño with a slice of bacon and secure with toothpicks.

Bake for 15 minutes or until bacon is crispy.

---

6. Avocado Tuna Salad

Net Carbs: 3g
Prep Time: 10 minutes
Style: Fresh
Cook Time: 0 minutes
Difficulty: Easy
No. Of SERVINGS: 2

INGREDIENTS:
- 1 avocado (diced)
- 1 can tuna (drained)
- 1/4 cup red onion (finely chopped)
- 1/4 cup celery (finely chopped)
- 2 tablespoons mayonnaise

- Add Salt and pepper to taste

DIRECTIONS:
In a bowl, mix diced avocado, drained tuna, red onion, celery, mayonnaise, salt, and pepper.
Serve as is or on cucumber slices.

---

7. Parmesan Crisps

Net Carbs: 1g
Prep Time: 10 minutes
Style: Baked
Cook Time: 8 minutes
Difficulty: Easy
No. Of SERVINGS: 4

INGREDIENTS:
- 1 cup shredded Parmesan cheese
- 1 teaspoon Italian seasoning
- 1/2 teaspoon garlic powder

DIRECTIONS:

Preheat the oven to 400°F (200°C).

Line a baking sheet with parchment paper.

Mix Parmesan cheese, Italian seasoning, and garlic powder.

Spoon small mounds onto the prepared baking sheet.

Bake for 8 minutes or until golden and crisp.

---

8. Guacamole Stuffed Mini Peppers

Net Carbs: 4g

Prep Time: 15 minutes

Style: Fresh

Cook Time: 0 minutes

Difficulty: Easy

No. Of SERVINGS: 4

INGREDIENTS:

- 12 mini bell peppers (halved and seeded)
- 2 avocados (mashed)

- 1 tomato (diced)
- 1/4 cup red onion (finely chopped)
- 1/4 cup cilantro (chopped)
- Lime juice, salt, and pepper to taste

DIRECTIONS:

In a bowl, mix mashed avocados, diced tomato, red onion, cilantro, lime juice, salt, and pepper.

Fill each mini pepper half with guacamole.

---

9. Greek Yogurt and Berry Parfait

Net Carbs: 5g
Prep Time: 10 minutes
Style: Fresh
Cook Time: 0 minutes
Difficulty: Easy
No. Of SERVINGS: 2

INGREDIENTS:

- 1 cup Greek yogurt (unsweetened)
- 1/2 cup mixed berries (strawberries, blueberries, raspberries)
- 2 tablespoons chopped nuts (almonds, walnuts)
- 1 tablespoon chia seeds
- Drizzle of sugar-free syrup

DIRECTIONS:

In a glass, layer Greek yogurt, mixed berries, chopped nuts, and chia seeds.
Drizzle with sugar-free syrup.
Repeat layers and enjoy.

---

10. Buffalo Cauliflower Bites

Net Carbs: 5g
Prep Time: 15 minutes
Style: Baked
Cook Time: 25 minutes
Difficulty: Moderate
No. Of SERVINGS: 4

INGREDIENTS:
- 1 head cauliflower (cut into florets)
- 1/2 cup buffalo sauce
- 1/4 cup melted butter
- 1 teaspoon garlic powder
- 1 teaspoon onion powder
- Ranch dressing for dipping

DIRECTIONS:
Preheat the oven to 450°F (230°C).
In a bowl, whisk buffalo sauce, melted butter, garlic powder, and onion powder.
Toss cauliflower florets in the buffalo sauce mixture.
Bake for 25 minutes or until crispy. Serve with ranch dressing.

11. Smoked Salmon Cucumber Rolls

Net Carbs: 1g
Prep Time: 10 minutes
Style: Fresh
Cook Time: 0 minutes
Difficulty: Easy
No. Of SERVINGS: 4

INGREDIENTS:
- 1 cucumber (sliced lengthwise)
- 4 oz smoked salmon
- Cream cheese
- Capers for garnish
- Fresh dill for garnish

DIRECTIONS:
Spread cream cheese on cucumber slices.
Place a strip of smoked salmon on each slice.
Roll the cucumber and salmon together.
Garnish with capers and fresh dill.

12. Keto Deviled Eggs

Net Carbs: 1g
Prep Time: 15 minutes
Style: Fresh
Cook Time: 15 minutes (for boiling eggs)
Difficulty: Easy
No. Of SERVINGS: 6

INGREDIENTS:
- 6 hard-boiled eggs (sliced in half)
- 2 tablespoons mayonnaise
- 1 teaspoon Dijon mustard
- Paprika and chives for garnish

DIRECTIONS:
Remove yolks from boiled eggs and mix with mayonnaise and Dijon mustard.
Spoon or pipe the yolk mixture back into the egg whites.
Garnish with paprika and chives.

13. Turkey and Cheese Roll-Ups

Net Carbs: 1g
Prep Time: 10 minutes
Style: Fresh
Cook Time: 0 minutes
Difficulty: Easy
No. Of SERVINGS: 4

INGREDIENTS:
- Deli turkey slices
- Cream cheese
- Pickle spears

DIRECTIONS:
Spread cream cheese on turkey slices.
Place a pickle spear at one end and roll up the turkey.
Then Secure with toothpicks if needed.

14: Spinach and Feta Stuffed Mushrooms

Net Carbs: 3g
Prep Time: 15 minutes
Style: Baked
Cook Time: 20 minutes
Difficulty: Moderate
No. Of SERVINGS: 4

INGREDIENTS:

- 12 large mushrooms (cleaned and stems removed)
- 1 cup spinach (chopped)
- 1/2 cup feta cheese (crumbled)
- 2 cloves garlic (minced)
- Olive oil for drizzling
- Salt and pepper to taste

DIRECTIONS:

Preheat the oven to 375°F (190°C).
In a skillet, sauté spinach, garlic, and feta until spinach wilts.

Stuff each mushroom cap with the spinach and feta mixture.

Drizzle with olive oil, season with salt and pepper, and bake for 20 minutes.

---

15. Keto Jalapeño Cheese Crisps

Net Carbs: 1g
Prep Time: 10 minutes
Style: Baked
Cook Time: 8 minutes
Difficulty: Easy
No. Of SERVINGS: 4

INGREDIENTS:
- 1 cup shredded cheddar cheese
- 1 jalapeño (sliced)
- 1 teaspoon garlic powder

DIRECTIONS:
Preheat the oven to 400°F (200°C).
Line a baking sheet with parchment paper.

Arrange small mounds of shredded cheddar cheese on the paper.
Top each mound with a jalapeño slice and sprinkle with garlic powder.
Bake for 8 minutes or until the edges are golden and crisp.

Atkins diet book

SALAD RECIPES

1. Buffalo Chicken Salad Recipe

Net Carbs 9.7 grams
Prep Time: 0 Minutes
Style:American
Cook Time: 45 Minutes
Difficulty: Difficult
2 Servings

INGREDIENTS

- 1/2 fruit (2-1/8" diameter) Lemon
- 1 medium (4-1/8" long) Young Green Onions
- 1/4 cup Real Mayonnaise
- 2 tablespoons Sour Cream
- 2/3 ounce Blue Cheese
- 1/8 teaspoon Garlic Powder
- 1 head Cos or Romaine Lettuce
- 2 stalk, medium (7-1/2" - 8" long) Celery
- 1 medium (approx 2-3/4" long, 2-1/2" diameter) Red Sweet Pepper

- 1 medium Tomato
- 1 large Egg
- 5 1/3 tablespoons Apple Cider Vinegar
- 1/4 cup Olive Oil
- 1/3 teaspoon Salt
- 1/4 teaspoon Black Pepper
- 1/8 teaspoon Celery Salt
- 1/8 teaspoon Red or Cayenne Pepper
- 2 thigh, bone removed Chicken Thigh Meat and Skin (Broilers or Fryers)

DIRECTIONS

Preheat the oven to 450°F and line a sheet pan with foil. In a large bowl, juice the lemon, remove the seeds, and finely chop the onions. Add mayonnaise, sour cream, blue cheese, and garlic powder to the lemon juice; stir to combine and set aside.

Prepare the vegetables: cut romaine into 1-inch pieces, celery into ½-inch pieces on a bias, slice red pepper into ¼-inch strips, and dice tomato into 1-inch pieces. Place all vegetables in the large bowl with the dressing (without tossing) and refrigerate until needed.

In a medium bowl, whisk the egg with a fork. Add apple cider vinegar, olive oil, salt, pepper, celery salt, and cayenne pepper. Whisk until well combined and frothy.

Pat each chicken thigh dry with a paper towel, dip in the egg mixture, and place on the prepared sheet pan. Bake for 18-20 minutes, turning thighs and brushing with the egg mixture several times until cooked through and crisp. Cut the chicken into ½-inch pieces.

Remove the salad from the refrigerator, toss the vegetables in the dressing, and divide between two plates. Top each plate with half the chicken and enjoy!

2. Grilled Chicken Caesar Salad

Net Carbs: 5 grams
Prep Time: 15 minutes
Style: Grilled
Cook Time:15 minutes
Difficulty: Easy
No. Of Servings: 4

INGREDIENTS:
- 4 boneless, skinless chicken breasts
- Romaine lettuce
- Parmesan cheese, grated
- Caesar dressing (low-carb)

INSTRUCTIONS:
Season chicken breasts with salt and pepper.
Grill chicken until cooked through.
Slice grilled chicken and place on a bed of Romaine lettuce.
Sprinkle with Parmesan cheese and drizzle with Caesar dressing.

3. Caprese Chicken Salad

Net Carbs: 4 grams
Prep Time: 15 minutes
Style:Italian-Inspired
Cook Time: 20 minutes
Difficulty: Easy
No. Of Servings: 2

INGREDIENTS:

- 2 boneless, skinless chicken breasts
- 1 cup cherry tomatoes, halved
- Fresh mozzarella, sliced
- Fresh basil leaves
- Balsamic glaze (low-carb)

INSTRUCTIONS:

Grill or bake chicken breasts until fully cooked.
Slice chicken and arrange on a plate.
Top with cherry tomatoes, mozzarella slices, and fresh basil.

Drizzle with balsamic glaze.

---

4. Classic Cobb Salad

Net Carbs: 6g
Prep Time: 15 minutes
Style: Fresh
Cook Time: 0 minutes
Difficulty: Easy
No. Of SERVINGS: 2

INGREDIENTS:

- 2 cups mixed salad greens
- 6 oz grilled chicken breast (sliced)
- 2 boiled eggs (sliced)
- 1 avocado (diced)
- 1/2 cup cherry tomatoes (halved)
- 1/4 cup blue cheese (crumbled)
- Bacon bits
- Ranch dressing

DIRECTIONS:

Arrange salad greens on a plate.

Top with sliced chicken, boiled eggs, diced avocado, cherry tomatoes, blue cheese, and bacon bits.

Drizzle with ranch dressing.

---

5. Spinach and Mushroom Salad

Net Carbs: 4g
Prep Time: 10 minutes
Style: Fresh
Cook Time: 0 minutes
Difficulty: Easy
No. Of SERVINGS: 4

INGREDIENTS:
- 6 cups fresh spinach
- 1 cup mushrooms (sliced)
- 1/4 cup red onion (thinly sliced)
- 1/4 cup feta cheese (crumbled)
- 1/4 cup toasted pine nuts

- Balsamic vinaigrette

DIRECTIONS:
In a large bowl, combine fresh spinach, sliced mushrooms, red onion, feta cheese, and toasted pine nuts.
Toss with balsamic vinaigrette before serving.

---

6. Grilled Shrimp and Avocado Salad

Net Carbs: 5g
Prep Time: 20 minutes
Style: Grilled
Cook Time: 5 minutes
Difficulty: Easy
No. Of SERVINGS: 3

INGREDIENTS:
- 1 lb shrimp (peeled and deveined)
- 2 tablespoons olive oil
- 1 teaspoon paprika

- Salt and pepper to taste
- 6 cups mixed salad greens
- 1 avocado (sliced)
- Cherry tomatoes
- Cucumber slices
- Lemon vinaigrette

DIRECTIONS:
Toss shrimp with olive oil, paprika, salt, and pepper. Grill until cooked.
Arrange salad greens on a plate, top with grilled shrimp, avocado slices, cherry tomatoes, and cucumber slices.
Drizzle with lemon vinaigrette.

---

7. Caesar Salad with Grilled Chicken

Net Carbs: 4g
Prep Time: 15 minutes
Style: Grilled
Cook Time: 15 minutes
Difficulty: Easy

No. Of SERVINGS: 2

INGREDIENTS:
- 2 boneless, skinless chicken breasts
- 2 tablespoons olive oil
- 1 teaspoon garlic powder
- Salt and pepper to taste
- 8 cups romaine lettuce (chopped)
- 1/2 cup grated Parmesan cheese
- Caesar dressing

DIRECTIONS:
Rub chicken with olive oil, garlic powder, salt, and pepper. Grill until cooked.
Chop grilled chicken and toss with chopped romaine and Parmesan cheese.
Drizzle with Caesar dressing before serving.

8. Caprese Salad

Net Carbs: 4g
Prep Time: 10 minutes
Style: Fresh
Cook Time: 0 minutes
Difficulty: Easy
No. Of SERVINGS: 4

INGREDIENTS:
- 4 large tomatoes (sliced)
- 1 lb fresh mozzarella cheese (sliced)
- Fresh basil leaves
- Balsamic glaze
- Olive oil
- Salt and pepper to taste

DIRECTIONS:
Arrange tomato and mozzarella slices on a platter, alternating and overlapping.
Put fresh basil leaves between tomato and mozzarella slices.

Drizzle with balsamic glaze and olive oil. Season with salt and pepper.

---

9. Tuna and Avocado Salad

Net Carbs: 3g
Prep Time: 15 minutes
Style: Fresh
Cook Time: 0 minutes
Difficulty: Easy
No. Of SERVINGS: 3

INGREDIENTS:
- 2 cans tuna (drained)
- 1 avocado (diced)
- 1/4 cup red onion (finely chopped)
- 1/4 cup celery (finely chopped)
- 2 tablespoons mayonnaise
- Lemon juice, salt, and pepper to taste
- Mixed salad greens

DIRECTIONS:
In a bowl, mix drained tuna, diced avocado, red onion, celery, mayonnaise, lemon juice, salt, and pepper.
Serve over mixed salad greens.

---

10. Greek Salad

Net Carbs: 5g
Prep Time: 15 minutes
Style: Fresh
Cook Time: 0 minutes
Difficulty: Easy
No. Of SERVINGS: 4

INGREDIENTS:
- 4 cups mixed salad greens
- 1 cucumber (sliced)
- 1 cup cherry tomatoes (halved)
- 1/2 cup Kalamata olives
- 1/2 cup feta cheese (crumbled)
- Red onion (thinly sliced)
- Greek dressing

DIRECTIONS:

In a large bowl, combine salad greens, sliced cucumber, cherry tomatoes, Kalamata olives, crumbled feta, and sliced red onion. Toss with Greek dressing before serving.

---

11. Steak and Blue Cheese Salad

Net Carbs: 6g
Prep Time: 20 minutes
Style: Grilled
Cook Time: 10 minutes
Difficulty: Moderate
No. Of SERVINGS: 2

INGREDIENTS:
- 1 lb sirloin steak
- 2 tablespoons olive oil
- Salt and pepper to taste
- 8 cups mixed salad greens
- 1/2 cup cherry tomatoes (halved)
- 1/4 cup red onion (thinly sliced)

- 1/4 cup blue cheese (crumbled)
- Balsamic vinaigrette

DIRECTIONS:
Rub steak with olive oil, salt, and pepper. Grill until desired doneness.
Slice grilled steak and arrange on mixed salad greens.
Top with cherry tomatoes, sliced red onion, and crumbled blue cheese.
Drizzle with balsamic vinaigrette.

---

12. Broccoli and Bacon Salad

Net Carbs: 5g
Prep Time: 15 minutes
Style: Fresh
Cook Time: 0 minutes
Difficulty: Easy
No. Of SERVINGS: 4

INGREDIENTS:

- 4 cups broccoli florets (blanched)
- 1/2 cup cooked bacon (crumbled)
- 1/4 cup red onion (finely chopped)
- 1/2 cup cheddar cheese (shredded)
- 1/4 cup mayonnaise
- 2 tablespoons apple cider vinegar
- 1 tablespoon erythritol (optional)
- Salt and pepper to taste

DIRECTIONS:

In a large bowl, combine blanched broccoli, crumbled bacon, chopped red onion, and shredded cheddar cheese.

In a small bowl, whisk together mayonnaise, apple cider vinegar, erythritol (if using), salt, and pepper.

Pour the dressing over the broccoli mixture and toss to combine.

13. Chicken and Strawberry Salad

Net Carbs: 6g
Prep Time: 15 minutes
Style: Fresh
Cook Time: 10 minutes (for chicken)
Difficulty: Easy
No. Of SERVINGS: 2

INGREDIENTS:
- 2 boneless, skinless chicken breasts
- 2 tablespoons olive oil
- Salt and pepper to taste
- 8 cups mixed salad greens
- 1 cup strawberries (sliced)
- 1/4 cup feta cheese (crumbled)
- Balsamic vinaigrette

DIRECTIONS:
Rub chicken with olive oil, salt, and pepper. Grill until cooked.
Slice grilled chicken and arrange on mixed salad greens.

Top with sliced strawberries and crumbled feta.

Drizzle with balsamic vinaigrette.

---

14. Asparagus and Goat Cheese Salad

Net Carbs: 4g
Prep Time: 15 minutes
Style: Grilled
Cook Time: 10 minutes
Difficulty: Easy
No. Of SERVINGS: 4

INGREDIENTS:
1 lb asparagus (trimmed)
2 tablespoons olive oil
Add Salt and pepper to taste
6 cups mixed salad greens
1/2 cup cherry tomatoes (halved)
1/4 cup goat cheese (crumbled)
Lemon vinaigrette

DIRECTIONS:

Toss asparagus with olive oil, salt, and pepper. Grill until tender.

Arrange mixed salad greens on a plate, top with grilled asparagus, cherry tomatoes, and crumbled goat cheese.

Drizzle with lemon vinaigrette.

---

15. Shrimp and Mango Salad

Net Carbs: 5g
Prep Time: 20 minutes
Style: Fresh
Cook Time: 5 minutes
Difficulty: Easy
No. Of SERVINGS: 3

INGREDIENTS:

- 1 lb shrimp (peeled and deveined)
- 1 tablespoon olive oil
- 1 teaspoon chili powder
- Add Salt and pepper to taste
- 6 cups mixed salad greens

- 1 mango (diced)
- 1/4 cup red onion (thinly sliced)
- Cilantro for garnish
- Lime vinaigrette

DIRECTIONS:
Toss shrimp with olive oil, chili powder, salt, and pepper. Grill until cooked.

Arrange mixed salad greens on a plate, top with grilled shrimp, diced mango, and sliced red onion.

Garnish with cilantro and drizzle with lime vinaigrette.

---

16. Egg and Bacon Spinach Salad

Net Carbs: 4g
Prep Time: 15 minutes
Style: Fresh
Cook Time: 10 minutes (for eggs and bacon)
Difficulty: Easy
No. Of SERVINGS: 4

INGREDIENTS:
- 8 cups fresh spinach
- 4 hard-boiled eggs (sliced)
- 1/2 cup cooked bacon (crumbled)
- 1/4 cup red onion (thinly sliced)
- 1/4 cup feta cheese (crumbled)
- Dijon vinaigrette

DIRECTIONS:

Arrange fresh spinach on a platter, top with sliced hard-boiled eggs, crumbled bacon, sliced red onion, and crumbled feta.

Drizzle with Dijon vinaigrette before serving.

---

17. Turkey and Cranberry Salad

Net Carbs: 5g
Prep Time: 15 minutes
Style: Fresh
Cook Time: 0 minutes
Difficulty: Easy
No. Of SERVINGS: 3

INGREDIENTS:

- 2 cups cooked turkey (shredded)
- 1/2 cup cranberries (fresh or dried)
- 1/4 cup pecans (chopped)
- 6 cups mixed salad greens
- 1/4 cup blue cheese (crumbled)
- Balsamic vinaigrette

DIRECTIONS:

In a large bowl, combine shredded turkey, cranberries, chopped pecans, mixed salad greens, and crumbled blue cheese.

Toss with balsamic vinaigrette before serving.

SMOOTHIE RECIPES

1. Golden Milk Chai Shake Smoothie Recipe

Net Carbs 3.6 grams
Prep Time: 5 Minutes
Method: Indian
Cooking Time: 0 Minutes
Difficulty: Easy
1 Serving

INGREDIENTS
- 1 shake Atkins Chai Tea Latte Protein Shake
- 2 tablespoons canned coconut milk
- 1/2 teaspoon turmeric, ground
- 1/4 teaspoon fresh ginger root

DIRECTIONS
Chill shake in the freezer for about 40 to 45 minutes from room temperature, or about 25 to 30 minutes from refrigerated.

Blend all ingredients together on medium high speed until well combined. Serve immediately over ice if desired.

---

2. Berry Almond Smoothie

Net Carbs: 6g
Prep Time: 5 minutes
Style: Blended
Difficulty: Easy
No. Of SERVINGS: 1

INGREDIENTS:
- 1/2 cup mixed berries (strawberries, blueberries, raspberries)
- 1/4 cup almond butter
- 1 cup unsweetened almond milk
- 1 tablespoon chia seeds
- Ice cubes

DIRECTIONS:
In a blender, combine mixed berries, almond butter, almond milk, and chia seeds.

Blend until smooth.
Add ice cubes and blend again until desired consistency.

---

3. Avocado Spinach Green Smoothie

Net Carbs: 5g
Prep Time: 7 minutes
Style: Blended
Difficulty: Easy
No. Of SERVINGS: 1

INGREDIENTS:
- 1/2 avocado
- 1 cup fresh spinach
- 1/2 cucumber (peeled and sliced)
- 1/2 lemon (juiced)
- 1 cup coconut water
- Stevia or erythritol to taste
- Ice cubes

DIRECTIONS:
Combine avocado, spinach, cucumber, lemon juice, coconut water, and sweetener in a blender.
Blend until smooth.
Add ice cubes and blend again for a refreshing green smoothie.

---

4. Chocolate Peanut Butter Protein Smoothie

Net Carbs: 4g
Prep Time: 5 minutes
Style: Blended
Difficulty: Easy
No. Of SERVINGS: 1

INGREDIENTS:
- 1 scoop chocolate protein powder
- 2 tablespoons peanut butter
- 1 cup unsweetened almond milk

- 1/2 teaspoon vanilla extract
- Ice cubes

DIRECTIONS:
In a blender, combine chocolate protein powder, peanut butter, almond milk, and vanilla extract.
Blend until well mixed.
Add ice cubes and blend again for a creamy chocolate peanut butter treat.

---

5. Coconut Berry Bliss Smoothie

Net Carbs: 7g
Prep Time: 6 minutes
Style: Blended
Difficulty: Easy
No. Of SERVINGS: 1

INGREDIENTS:
- 1/2 cup mixed berries (strawberries, blueberries, raspberries)
- 1/2 cup coconut cream

- 1/2 cup unsweetened coconut milk
- 1 tablespoon chia seeds
- 1 teaspoon coconut oil
- Ice cubes

DIRECTIONS:

Blend mixed berries, coconut cream, coconut milk, chia seeds, and coconut oil until smooth.

Add ice cubes and blend for a refreshing and tropical coconut berry smoothie.

---

6. Vanilla Almond Butter Smoothie

Net Carbs: 5g
Prep Time: 5 minutes
Style: Blended
Phase: Ongoing Weight Loss (OWL)
Difficulty: Easy
No. Of SERVINGS: 1

INGREDIENTS:

- 1 cup unsweetened almond milk
- 1 scoop vanilla protein powder
- 2 tablespoons almond butter
- 1/2 teaspoon cinnamon
- Stevia or erythritol to taste
- Ice cubes

DIRECTIONS:

Blend almond milk, vanilla protein powder, almond butter, cinnamon, and sweetener until creamy.

Add ice cubes and blend again for a smooth and satisfying vanilla almond butter smoothie.

---

7. Green Apple Ginger Zinger Smoothie

Net Carbs: 6g
Prep Time: 8 minutes
Style: Blended
Difficulty: Easy

No. Of SERVINGS: 1

INGREDIENTS:
- 1 green apple (cored and sliced)
- 1 cup kale leaves (stems removed)
- 1/2 inch fresh ginger (peeled)
- 1/2 lemon (juiced)
- 1 cup unsweetened almond milk
- Stevia or erythritol to taste
- Ice cubes

DIRECTIONS:
Blend green apple, kale, ginger, lemon juice, almond milk, and sweetener until smooth. Add ice cubes and blend again for a refreshing green apple ginger zinger.

---

8. Blueberry Avocado Dream Smoothie

Net Carbs: 7g
Prep Time: 6 minutes
Style: Blended

Difficulty: Easy
No. Of SERVINGS: 1

INGREDIENTS:

- 1/2 cup blueberries
- 1/2 avocado
- 1/2 cup Greek yogurt (unsweetened)
- 1 tablespoon flax seeds
- 1 cup almond milk
- Stevia or erythritol to taste
- Ice cubes

DIRECTIONS:

Blend blueberries, avocado, Greek yogurt, flaxseeds, almond milk, and sweetener until creamy.

Add ice cubes and blend again for a luscious blueberry avocado dream.

9. Cinnamon Spice Pumpkin Smoothie

Net Carbs: 6g
Prep Time: 7 minutes
Style: Blended
Difficulty: Easy
No. Of SERVINGS: 1

INGREDIENTS:

- 1/2 cup canned pumpkin (unsweetened)
- 1/2 teaspoon cinnamon
- 1/4 teaspoon nutmeg
- 1 cup unsweetened coconut milk
- 1 scoop vanilla protein powder
- Stevia or erythritol to taste
- Ice cubes

DIRECTIONS:

Blend canned pumpkin, cinnamon, nutmeg, coconut milk, vanilla protein powder, and sweetener until smooth.

Add ice cubes and blend for a delightful cinnamon spice pumpkin smoothie.

---

10. Mango Coconut Delight Smoothie

Net Carbs: 8g
Prep Time: 5 minutes
Style: Blended
Difficulty: Easy
No. Of SERVINGS: 1

INGREDIENTS:

- 1/2 cup mango chunks
- 1/2 cup coconut cream
- 1/2 cup unsweetened coconut milk
- 1 tablespoon chia seeds
- 1 teaspoon lime juice
- Stevia or erythritol to taste
- Ice cubes

DIRECTIONS:

Blend mango chunks, coconut cream, coconut milk, chia seeds, lime juice, and sweetener until creamy.
Add ice cubes and blend again for a tropical mango coconut delight.

---

11. Strawberry Basil Bliss Smoothie

Net Carbs: 6g
Prep Time: 8 minutes
Style: Blended
Difficulty: Easy
No. Of SERVINGS: 1

INGREDIENTS:

- 1/2 cup strawberries
- 5-6 fresh basil leaves
- 1/2 cup Greek yogurt (unsweetened)
- 1 tablespoon hemp seeds
- 1 cup unsweetened almond milk
- Stevia or erythritol to taste
- Ice cubes

DIRECTIONS:
Blend strawberries, basil leaves, Greek yogurt, hemp seeds, almond milk, and sweetener until smooth.
Add ice cubes and blend for a refreshing strawberry basil bliss.

---

12. Peanut Butter Banana Power Smoothie

Net Carbs: 7g
Prep Time: 6 minutes
Style: Blended
Difficulty: Easy
No. Of SERVINGS: 1

INGREDIENTS:
- 1/2 banana
- 2 tablespoons peanut butter
- 1 scoop chocolate protein powder
- 1 cup unsweetened almond milk
- 1 tablespoon chia seeds

- Stevia or erythritol to taste
- Ice cubes

DIRECTIONS:
Blend banana, peanut butter, chocolate protein powder, almond milk, chia seeds, and sweetener until creamy.
Add ice cubes and blend again for a power-packed peanut butter banana smoothie.

---

13. Kiwi Kale Citrus Smoothie

Net Carbs: 6g
Prep Time: 7 minutes
Style: Blended
Difficulty: Easy
No. Of SERVINGS: 1

INGREDIENTS:
- 2 kiwis (peeled and sliced)
- 1 cup kale leaves (stems removed)
- 1/2 orange (peeled)

- 1/2 lemon (juiced)
- 1 cup coconut water
- Stevia or erythritol to taste
- Ice cubes

DIRECTIONS:
Blend kiwis, kale, orange, lemon juice, coconut water, and sweetener until smooth. Add ice cubes and blend for a zesty kiwi kale citrus smoothie.

---

14. Raspberry Coconut Chia Smoothie

Net Carbs: 7g
Prep Time: 6 minutes
Style: Blended
Difficulty: Easy
No. Of SERVINGS: 1

INGREDIENTS:
- 1/2 cup raspberries
- 1/2 cup coconut milk

- 1 tablespoon chia seeds
- 1/2 teaspoon vanilla extract
- 1 tablespoon unsweetened shredded coconut
- Stevia or erythritol to taste
- Ice cubes

DIRECTIONS:
Blend raspberries, coconut milk, chia seeds, vanilla extract, shredded coconut, and sweetener until creamy.
Add ice cubes and blend for a luscious raspberry coconut chia smoothie.

---

15. Coffee Almond Protein Smoothie

Net Carbs: 5g
Prep Time: 5 minutes
Style: Blended
Difficulty: Easy
No. Of SERVINGS: 1

INGREDIENTS:

- 1/2 cup brewed coffee (cooled)
- 1 scoop vanilla protein powder
- 2 tablespoons almond butter
- 1 cup unsweetened almond milk
- 1/2 teaspoon cinnamon
- Stevia or erythritol to taste
- Ice cubes

DIRECTIONS:

In a blender, combine brewed coffee, vanilla protein powder, almond butter, almond milk, cinnamon, and sweetener.
Blend until smooth.
Add ice cubes and blend again for a caffeinated coffee almond protein boost.

---

16. Pineapple Mint Green Smoothie

Net Carbs: 8g
Prep Time: 7 minutes
Style: Blended
Difficulty: Easy
No. Of SERVINGS: 1

INGREDIENTS:

- 1/2 cup pineapple chunks
- Handful of fresh mint leaves
- 1/2 cucumber (peeled and sliced)
- 1/2 lime (juiced)
- 1 cup spinach leaves
- 1 cup coconut water
- Stevia or erythritol to taste
- Ice cubes

DIRECTIONS:

Blend pineapple chunks, mint leaves, cucumber, lime juice, spinach leaves, coconut water, and sweetener until refreshing.

Add ice cubes and blend again for a tropical pineapple mint green smoothie.

TIPS AND TRICKS

GROCERY SHOPPING FOR ATKINS DIET.

As individual needs may vary, consulting with a healthcare professional or a nutritionist can provide personalized guidance for your specific health goals and requirements. So when grocery shopping for the Atkins diet, here i made a brief list of 12 ultimate tips and tricks to help you make informed and better choices:

Focus on Whole Foods:
Prioritize fresh, whole foods like vegetables, fruits (in moderation), meat, poultry, fish, eggs, and dairy.

Check Nutritional Labels:
Pay attention to nutritional labels to identify the carb content of packaged items. Look for products with lower net carbs.

Choose Healthy Fats:
Opt for healthy fats like avocados, olive oil, coconut oil, and nuts. These provide satiety and are essential for a low-carb, high-fat diet.

Stock Up on Low-Carb Vegetables:
Load your cart with low-carb vegetables such as leafy greens, broccoli, cauliflower, zucchini, and bell peppers.

Select Lean Proteins:
Choose lean protein sources like chicken, turkey, fish, and lean cuts of beef or pork. Protein is a crucial component of the Atkins diet.

Explore Sugar Substitutes:
Look for sugar substitutes like stevia or erythritol for sweetening without adding extra carbs.

Include Dairy:

Incorporate low-carb dairy options such as cheese, butter, and unsweetened almond or coconut milk.

Plan Ahead:

Plan your meals for the week and create a shopping list. This helps you stay focused on your dietary goals and avoids impulsive purchases.

Avoid Processed Carbs:

Steer clear of processed and refined carbs, including sugary snacks, pastries, and most grains.

Explore Specialty Sections:

Check out specialty sections for low-carb products, such as almond flour, coconut flour, and sugar-free condiments.

Shop Online:

Consider online shopping for specialty low-carb items and a wider variety of options.

Stay Hydrated:

Prioritize water and low-carb beverages. Avoid sugary drinks and high-carb beverages.

MEAL PLANNING AND PREPPING.

Meal planning and prepping are powerful tools to stay on track with your Atkins diet goals. Consider tailoring your approach to fit your schedule and preferences, and don't hesitate to experiment with new recipes and flavors.

Here are ultimate tips and tricks to make meal planning and prepping a breeze:

Create a Weekly Menu:

Plan your meals for the week ahead. This helps you organize your shopping list and ensures you have all the necessary ingredients.

Batch Cooking:

Cook in batches to save time during the week. Prepare larger quantities of proteins, vegetables, and other staples that can be used for multiple meals.

Variety is Key:

Ensure variety in your meals to avoid monotony. Explore different protein sources, vegetables, and cooking methods to keep your meals interesting.

Pre-cut and Wash Vegetables:**

Spend some time washing, chopping, and prepping vegetables in advance. Store them in containers for easy access when you're ready to cook.

Pre-Portion Snacks:

Pre-portion snacks like nuts, cheese, or veggies to avoid overeating and make it easy to grab a quick, satisfying snack.

Plan for Leftovers:

Plan meals that can double as leftovers. This minimizes cooking time on busy days and helps reduce food waste.

Invest in Storage Containers:

Invest in good-quality storage containers to keep your prepped meals fresh. Choose containers that are freezer-safe for longer storage.

Label and Date:

Label containers with the date of preparation to keep track of freshness. This is especially important when storing items in the freezer.

Prep Protein for Quick Meals:

Cook a variety of proteins (chicken, beef, fish) and keep them in the fridge. They can be easily incorporated into salads, stir-fries, or omelets.

Prepare Dressings and Sauces:

Make low-carb dressings and sauces in advance. Having these on hand can enhance the flavor of your meals without adding unnecessary carbs.

Keep Essentials Stocked:

Ensure you have Atkins-friendly essentials like olive oil, herbs, spices, and low-carb condiments stocked in your pantry.

Schedule Prep Time:

Dedicate a specific time each week for meal prep. Consistency makes the process more manageable and helps you stay organized.

Be Mindful of Portion Sizes:

When prepping meals, consider portion sizes to align with your dietary goals. This helps control calorie and carb intake.

Stay Flexible:

While planning is crucial, be flexible. Life can be unpredictable, so have backup options for quick and easy low-carb meals.

SUBSTITUTIONS FOR COMMON INGREDIENTS IN THE ATKINS DIET.

These substitutions mentioned below allow you to enjoy a variety of delicious meals while adhering to the principles of the Atkins diet. Always check labels and nutritional information to ensure that your substitutions align with your carb goals.

There are times you may need to make substitutions for common ingredients to keep your meals low in carbohydrates. I made a wonderful handy list down there for you.

Flour:

 Substitute almond flour or coconut flour for traditional wheat flour in recipes. These alternatives are lower in carbs and suitable for various baking needs.

Sugar:

Use sugar substitutes such as stevia, erythritol, or monk fruit sweetener instead of regular sugar. They add sweetness without the added carbs.

Bread:

Opt for low-carb bread alternatives like almond flour bread, coconut flour bread, or lettuce wraps instead of traditional bread.

Rice:

Replace rice with cauliflower rice. Simply grate or process cauliflower into rice-sized pieces and cook. It has a similar texture to rice but with fewer carbs.

Pasta:

Choose spiralized vegetables like zucchini or spaghetti squash as a substitute for pasta. They offer a satisfying noodle-like texture without the carb load.

Potatoes:

Use cauliflower as a low-carb substitute for potatoes. Mash or roast cauliflower for a similar texture without the high carbohydrate content.

Milk:

Opt for unsweetened almond milk, coconut milk, or cashew milk instead of regular cow's milk. These alternatives are lower in carbs and suitable for various recipes.

Cream:

Replace heavy cream with full-fat coconut milk or coconut cream. It provides a rich, creamy texture with fewer carbs.

Yogurt:

Choose Greek yogurt or coconut milk yogurt instead of traditional yogurt. Ensure they are unsweetened to keep the carb count low.

Cereal:

Make a low-carb cereal by mixing nuts, seeds, and unsweetened coconut flakes. Add almond milk for a satisfying and crunchy breakfast.

Snack Bars:

Make your own low-carb snack bars using ingredients like nuts, seeds, unsweetened coconut, and sugar substitutes. Check for suitable recipes online.

Crackers:

Opt for cheese crisps or flaxseed crackers as a low-carb alternative to traditional crackers.

Soy Sauce:

Choose tamari or coconut aminos instead of soy sauce. These alternatives are lower in carbs and suitable for those following a gluten-free diet.

Flavor Enhancers:

Experiment with herbs, spices, and low-carb condiments like mustard and hot sauce to add flavor without extra carbs.

CONCLUSION

RECAP OF THE ATKINS DIET PRINCIPLES

Following these principles, you can achieve weight loss, improved metabolic health, and long-term maintenance of a healthy lifestyle through the Atkins diet. It's essential to consult with a healthcare professional before making significant dietary changes.

Four Phases:
The Atkins diet consists of four phases: Induction, Ongoing Weight Loss (OWL), Pre-Maintenance, and Maintenance. Each phase has specific guidelines to gradually reintroduce carbs.

Low Carb, High Fat:
The diet emphasizes a low-carb, high-fat approach to encourage the body to burn fat for fuel, leading to weight loss.

Net Carbs:

Focus is on net carbs, which are total carbs minus fiber. Monitoring net carbs helps control blood sugar levels and supports ketosis.

Protein is Essential:

Adequate protein intake is encouraged to maintain muscle mass and support overall health.

Healthy Fats:

Emphasis on healthy fats, such as avocados, olive oil, and nuts, to provide sustained energy and promote satiety.

Phased Carbohydrate Introduction:

Carbohydrates are reintroduced gradually through the phases, allowing individuals to identify their tolerance levels without triggering weight gain.

Induction Phase (Phase 1):

Limits daily net carb intake to 20-25 grams to kickstart ketosis and initiate weight loss.

OWL Phase (Phase 2):

Gradually increases net carbs by introducing more vegetables and low-carb fruits while continuing weight loss.

Pre-Maintenance (Phase 3):

Further increases net carbs, allowing for a broader range of food choices. This phase prepares individuals for long-term weight maintenance.

Maintenance (Phase 4):

Focus on maintaining a healthy lifestyle with a balanced approach to carbohydrates. Individuals learn to sustain their weight loss while enjoying a variety of foods.

Hydration is Important:
Adequate hydration is encouraged throughout all phases of the diet.

Individualized Approach:
The Atkins diet acknowledges that individuals have different carb tolerances, and the approach can be customized based on personal preferences and health goals.

Regular Physical Activity:
Incorporating regular physical activity is encouraged for overall health and well-being.

Whole Foods Emphasis:
The diet promotes whole, unprocessed foods, including lean proteins, vegetables, and healthy fats.

Sugar & Processed Carbs Restriction:
Restriction of added sugars and processed carbohydrates is a key element to stabilize blood sugar levels.

ENCOURAGEMENT, MOTIVATION FOR SUCCESS & FINAL THOUGHTS

Encouragement:

Dear Atkins Warriors,

You've embarked on a journey to transform your life, embracing the principles of the Atkins diet. Remember, change takes time, and every small step you take is a victory. You are not just altering your eating habits; you are rewriting your relationship with food, carving a path to a healthier, more vibrant you.

Motivation for Success:

1. Celebrate Every Progress:

Whether it's a pound lost, a new healthy recipe conquered, or resisting that tempting dessert, celebrate each achievement. Small victories pave the way for significant success.

2. Fuel Your Body with Positivity:
Your journey is not just about physical transformation; it's a mental and emotional shift too. Fill your mind with positivity. You're not giving up your favorite foods; you're choosing a healthier, more fulfilling life.

3. Embrace the Learning Curve:
As you navigate the phases of Atkins, embrace the learning curve. Understand your body's response, discover what fuels you best, and relish the empowerment that comes with knowledge.

4. Stay Consistent, Not Perfect:
Consistency is your ally. It's not about perfection; it's about consistently making choices that align with your goals. Progress is progress, no matter how small.

5. You Are Worth It:
Remember, this journey is an investment in yourself. You are worth the effort, the

dedication, and the commitment. Keep envisioning the vibrant, healthier version of yourself.

Final Thoughts:

In the quiet moments of your journey, reflect on how far you've come. You are rewriting your story, creating a narrative of resilience, discipline, and self-love. The journey may have challenges, but each challenge is an opportunity to grow stronger.

As you savor the taste of success, relish in the fact that you are not just losing weight; you are gaining a life rich in health, vitality, and self-love. Trust the process, believe in yourself, and know that the decisions you make today are building the foundation for a healthier tomorrow.

With unwavering support,
Your Future Healthy Self.

Dear Reader,

I hope you enjoyed reading **Atkins Diet Book 2023 - 2024** **Rapid Weight Loss, Burn Fat, and the Simpler, Faster Path to a Low-Carb Lifestyle – Achieve Weight Loss Without Sacrifice**. I poured my heart and soul into researching and writing this book, and I would be so grateful if you could take a few minutes to share your thoughts with others. Your feedback is invaluable to me, and it can help me improve my writing and reach a wider audience. It also helps other readers decide whether or not they want to read my book.

Please consider leaving a review on Amazon, Goodreads, or any other platform where you purchased this book. Even a few sentences would be greatly appreciated. Thank you for your time and consideration.

Helen Munoz